THE STUDENT PARAMEDIC SURVIVAL GUIDE

Your Journey from Student to Paramedic

Amanda Y. Blaber

 Open University Press

Open University Press
McGraw-Hill Education
McGraw-Hill House
Shoppenhangers Road
Maidenhead
Berkshire
England
SL6 2QL

email: enquiries@openup.co.uk
world wide web: www.openup.co.uk

and Two Penn Plaza, New York, NY 10121–2289, USA

First published 2015

A catalogue record of this book is available from the British Library

ISBN-13: 978-0-335-26236-6 (pb)
ISBN-10: 0-335-26236-8 (pb)
eISBN: 978-0-335-26237-3

Library of Congress Cataloging-in-Publication Data
CIP data applied for

Typesetting and e-book compilations by
RefineCatch Limited, Bungay, Suffolk

Fictitious names of companies, products, people, characters and/or data that may be
used herein (in case studies or in examples) are not intended to represent any real
individual, company, product or event.

Printed and bound by CPI Group (UK) Ltd, Croydon, CR0 4YY

Praise for this book

"This is a must buy for any student from school leaver to the mature candidate who is thinking of studying to be a Paramedic. The book comprehensively addresses everything from where and how to apply, unpicking the complex picture of fees and funding to the realities of what to expect when you get to university and what it's like on placement. With valuable contributions from current students, academics and educators this book explains everything you need to know and might not have thought you needed to know before you apply."

Mark Nevins, Senior Lecturer, Teeside University, UK, and NMC Registered Adult Nurse and HCPC Registered Paramedic.

"I would consider this book as required reading for anyone considering embarking on a career as a paramedic. It is honest, informative and true to life. I liked the way that all aspects of student life were covered, from applications, to studying and placements and finally being out in the world.

This job isn't what a lot of people seem to think it is but Amanda has gone to great lengths to myth bust. This book shows a depth and consideration that all prospective paramedic students should appreciate. It is clear that a great deal of effort has gone into this survival guide."

Mark Young, Paramedic & Practice Placement Educator, South East Coast Ambulance Service, UK

"I liked the way that the book utilises a cross-section of students, practitioners and academics when providing opinions on the student paramedic journey, as this provides the triangulation required to ensure the views presented are representative of the student paramedic arena. It will provide a useful guide to the mysteries of the student journey. It is also useful that it illustrates the differences across the whole of the UK and considers the different approaches and how they can change the coping mechanisms that need to be used, and that are in place.

The 4 sections provide an excellent overview of the 4 areas that most student paramedics want to, and need to, know, and answers a number of the questions (if not all) asked very effectively. The sections also support the needs of the profession, as well as the

students own professional journey; covering a number of areas that are part of the institutional and ambulance Trusts inductions.

It is useful to note that The Survival Guide also recognises the differences the student paramedic experiences when compared to other students in universities. This means that the Survival Guide can act as an 'aide memoire' that is available when those difficult questions come up that need an immediate answer that can allay fears and anxieties and signpost the students to the places they can get support. This aspect is helped by the shared experiences from past and present students and practitioners, who act as mentors and paramedic educators to the students.

This book has been a long time coming and will, based on my experience, help the student to have a better transition towards their future professional role."

Lizzie Ryan, Education Business Manager and Clinical Training Manager (East) at South Western Ambulance Service NHS Foundation Trust, UK, also Lecturer at Bournemouth University, UK and Plymouth University, UK and the Open University, UK

For all student cohorts from 2004 to the present date.
Thanks to Amy, Carly, Joe, Rae and Marion Richardson.

CONTENTS

List of tables ix
List of authors and contributors x
How to use this book xiv
Introduction xvi

PART 1
Preparation for becoming a student paramedic 1

1 Is this the right career for me? 3

2 Choosing a programme and university 23

PART 2
Making the most of your academic study 39

3 How is paramedic academic study different from
other subjects? 41

4 What is a 'professional' programme? 76

5 What will I be studying? 95

6 Learning in simulation 107

7 How can I link my academic studies and
clinical practice? 118

PART 3
Placement: preparing for and making the most of it 123

8 Is practice what you think it is going to be? 125

9 What you wanted to do this for – the care of patients
and their families 140

10 What support is there when on placement? 151

11 Assessment in practice 164

12 Difficult cases 170

13 Resilience and support 177

14 Fitting in 191

PART 4
Transition to registration 195

15 Are you ready? 197

16 Getting your first job 205

17 Preceptorship 213

Conclusion 219
Index 220

LIST OF TABLES

2.1	Various levels of undergraduate study	24
2.2	Examples of the potential variation in fee status	31
2.3	Details of C1 driving category and blue-light driving course	35
3.1	The academic credit system	44
3.2	Activist characteristics and teaching activities	57
3.3	Reflector characteristics and teaching activities	58
3.4	Theorist characteristics and teaching activities	58
3.5	Pragmatist characteristics and teaching activities	59
3.6	Characteristics of visual learners	62
3.7	Characteristics of auditory learners	62
3.8	Characteristics of kinaesthetic learners	63
4.1	Guidance on conduct and ethics for students	82
5.1	Areas covered by the HCPC *Standards of Education and Training* (SETS)	96
5.2	College of Paramedics curriculum content categories	96
5.3	HCPC *Standards of Proficiency* for paramedics	97
8.1	Types of ambulance service placements that may be included in paramedic programmes	128
8.2	Types of non-ambulance service placements that may be included in paramedic programmes	133
10.1	SETs relating to support on practice placement	152
13.1	Sources of stress categorised into groups	178
13.2	The five dimensions of resilience in adults' lives	184
15.1	HCPC standards for CPD	203
16.1	Advice on preparing a supporting statement	208
16.2	Practical things you can do prior to interview	209
17.1	What preceptorship is not	215
17.2	Additional recommendations for the paramedic during the first six months following registration	217

LIST OF AUTHORS AND CONTRIBUTORS

Amanda Blaber MSc, PGDip HE, BSc(Hons), DipHE (A&E), RGN
Senior Lecturer, School of Health Sciences, University of Brighton

Prior to her career in education, Amanda worked in an emergency department where she taught, mentored student nurses and worked in partnership with ambulance staff for many years. Amanda has worked in three higher education institutions and has taught students on health care programmes since beginning her career in higher education in 2000. Amanda has been involved as programme and module leader, personal tutor, admissions and practice link tutor for paramedic programmes in all her higher education roles. Amanda has edited and co-edited several best-selling paramedic-specific textbooks. This text has been written by Amanda to better equip student paramedics for their personal, academic and clinical experiences within a paramedic programme. Amanda feels sure that the information within this text will empower students to make informed decisions that will enhance their journey to becoming a successful student and paramedic.

Kevin Barrett
Senior Lecturer, School of Health Sciences, University of Brighton

Kevin Barrett has been course leader for the BSc(Hons) in Paramedic Practice since 2009, and has long been involved in the development of clinical courses. Kevin is a registered nurse and was lecturer-practitioner for the Sussex Critical Care Network from 2003 to 2007. He recognises the value that simulation approaches have in the delivery of all areas of the curriculum and sees this as a rapidly developing area across health care. Simulation is becoming a key area in his own research interests, and he has written Chapter 6 of this book.

Paramedic students throughout the UK will meet simulated practice scenarios as they allow the rehearsal of complex and demanding elements of care in environments that are supportive of students' learning. It is a very useful preparation for those about to commence a paramedic course to be aware of the scope of possible simulation strategies that they might meet, how to prepare for engagement with these and the ways in which they encourage and develop the knowledge, skills and attitudes needed to register as a paramedic.

Gemma Chapman BSc(Hons) Paramedic Practice, MC Para, PPEd/PEd
Paramedic Operations Officer, South Western Ambulance Service NHS Foundation Trust

Gemma qualified as a paramedic in 2012 from the University of Brighton and worked initially for the South East Coast Ambulance Service NHS Foundation Trust, taking an active role in the selection and development of student paramedics. Gemma went on to complete her practice educator/mentorship module through the university before moving trusts to join the South Western Ambulance Service NHS Foundation Trust. Here Gemma worked solo on a rapid response vehicle before accepting a position as a paramedic operations officer, being responsible for providing clinical leadership and ensuring the day-to-day management of a group of stations whilst effectively leading operational staff to ensure delivery of high-quality patient care. Gemma is currently working towards an extended diploma in Leadership and Management. Having experienced the path from student to paramedic so recently, Gemma hopes that her passion and enthusiasm for a paramedic career shine through in the contributions she has made to the chapters of this book.

Sarah Christopher Dip PHC, BSc(Hons), PGCE LTHE, FHEA, MC Para
Senior Lecturer, Faculty of Health and Wellbeing, Sheffield Hallam University

Sarah joined the NHS ambulance service in 1996 and qualified as a paramedic in 1999. In addition to her paramedic registration she holds a first-class honours degree in Pre-Hospital Care, Royal College of Surgeons Medicine in Remote Areas and Travel and Tropical Health qualifications, Pre-Hospital Trauma Life Support, Intermediate Trauma Life Support and Post-Graduate Certificate in Learning and Teaching in Higher Education. She is a Fellow of the Higher Education Academy.

Whilst in the ambulance service she acted as clinical and academic support to student paramedics. She also worked in the private sector and on a technical rescue team in industry. She has had in excess of 20 articles published to date in a wide range of medical journals and hopes to begin studying towards a master's degree in Education in the near future.

She joined university full-time in September 2010 which enabled her to help and guide the paramedics of the future, something she feels very passionately about. She still keeps a contract for occasional work with East Midlands Ambulance Service.

Amy Hammerton BSc(Hons) Paramedic Practice, MC Para
Paramedic on relief rota in West Suffolk area of East of England Ambulance Service NHS Trust

Amy qualified as a paramedic in 2013. Amy's interest in the student paramedic and mentor/PEd roles began when she was a student paramedic at university. Amy experienced different attitudes of ambulance personnel towards students, predominantly from mentors/PEds. It was these experiences that led Amy to write her dissertation on the subject of mentorship within paramedicine. Amy is now 2 years post registration, as a paramedic, and has applied to be a mentor/PEd. Amy hopes to make students' experiences positive and fulfilling while actively taking part in shaping the future of the profession.

Marion Richardson BA(Hons), MA Education, MC Para
Programme leader for the BSc(Hons) Paramedic Practice programme in the School of Health at Teesside University

Marion is an HCPC registered paramedic and has a long history of delivering paramedic education within both the ambulance service and higher education. Marion spent most of her professional career in practice working as a paramedic and divisional education lead within the North East Ambulance Service. Marion joined Teesside University in 2009 and uses her practice experience to inform the teaching of student paramedics. She has had leadership responsibilities for a range of programmes including the Foundation Degree Paramedic Science programme, BSc(Hons) Paramedic Practice programme and a range of postgraduate modules. Marion is passionate about paramedic practice and education and has a particular interest in mentorship and preceptorship.

Christopher Storey BSc(Hons) Paramedic Practice, MC Para

Before becoming a paramedic Chris had a 17-year career as a Church minister and a five-year career as a learning support assistant (LSA) with disabled children and young people. One lunchtime at the school where Chris worked he was talking with one of the students who has a life-shortening condition. The student asked Chris what job he would love to do if he could (other than working as an LSA). Chris told him he had always secretly wished to become a paramedic, but at 45 felt too old to start the education and study involved. The student reminded Chris that, however old he was, he would still live longer than the student would and dared Chris to try and become a paramedic. Having accepted his challenge, Chris attended an access course in order to gain the qualifications needed to apply to university. Chris then gained a place at university. Three years later Chris graduated with a first-class honours degree and is now working as a paramedic for an ambulance trust.

Chris found that one of the most useful things at university was talking with other students who had already been through the programme. Their insight broadened Chris's understanding, helped prepare him for practice and enabled him to achieve more than he thinks he would have without it. Chris hopes the insights he has given in this book will do the same for any prospective students reading it.

HOW TO USE THIS BOOK

This book will provide you with a realistic view of the journey from student to paramedic. The information, comments, responses, case studies and reflection points offered will interest and may sometimes surprise you, but will leave you wanting to learn and investigate more. The intention is that this text will be a valuable resource from the initial consideration of your journey and throughout, to the culmination in the start of a successful career as a paramedic.

A variety of approaches have been taken in order to elicit useful and realistic information for the reader. The contributor profiles include student paramedics, academics, paramedics and paramedic mentors/paramedic educators (PEds). These contributors come from a variety of institutions and ambulance services covering many regions of England. This text is inclusive and useful for students studying towards paramedic registration across all areas of England, and the book will also be of use beyond this, in the rest of the United Kingdom.

In all chapters, within each part of this text, the contributors have had the freedom to make specific comments relating to the subject being discussed. Throughout the text there are sections that offer comments/responses to questions. The contributors are identified as follows:

    📖   denotes comments/responses to questions from students

    🔦   denotes responses to questions from paramedics and/or paramedic mentors/PEds

    🎓   denotes responses to questions from academics

The symbols will make the comments from the contributor easy to find and will enable readers to compare and contrast the views of each of them. Some of the comments are short, others have been summarised and some are longer, with greater explanation. For visual aesthetic reasons quotation marks have been removed. The 📖 symbol has been used for the student comments in Chapter 1, so it can be clearly seen that views have been voiced by many and not just one or two students. Some of the comments/responses to questions may contradict each other; this is not surprising, considering the different roles and experiences the contributors will have had. Some comments/responses to questions may be quite controversial and may present a different reality than that expected by the reader.

The contributors have been asked to respond to specific questions, and you will be able to read the question/s posed and the individual responses. In Chapter 1, the questions and responses have been collated from students in specific cohorts at various points in their academic studies. Their comments represent a wide range of views, some conflicting, and as unique as each individual student, in order to provide the reader with the diversity of opinion based on experience.

The intention is that many of the comments will encourage you to think more deeply about aspects of your study and practice. This text will endeavour to present a realistic view within its chapters, and in some areas may challenge your assumptions and impressions, with regard to studying in a higher education environment and working in a clinical environment.

Throughout this text anonymity is maintained, names used are pseudonyms, and all experiences recalled and commented on have been adapted and are included for illustrative purposes only.

In addition, there are:

- case studies
- sections linked to each other; for easy cross-referencing
- reflection points
- suggested reading for each chapter.

INTRODUCTION

Embarking on a new journey, in the form of a different or new career move, could make a significant change to your life. Whatever your individual journey, your decision to want to become a paramedic is not one that can be taken lightly. This career may be something you have worked towards whilst at school or college. However, for some it will be a change of career and re-entry into higher education.

This text is the culmination of relevant student and professionals' experiences as they have reflected on their own journeys to becoming a paramedic. The text specifically includes the comments, thoughts and suggestions of students and colleagues from the practice and academic environment.

The said contributors aim to bring you, the reader, some of their *pearls of wisdom* from reality, in order that you can be as prepared as possible for your academic and professional journey towards your career as a paramedic. The cross-section of students (junior and senior), paramedics, paramedic mentors/paramedic educators (PEds) and academics making comments throughout the text represent a wide geographical area, variety of higher education institutes and ambulance trusts. By adopting this inclusive approach, the text will be largely representative of the educational and clinical practice experiences of students across England. There are some variations across Scotland, Wales and Northern and Southern Ireland in respect of the types of programmes offered (both higher education institution and ambulance service in-house routes in some areas). These differences also encompass funding, and specific guidance should be sought from the region concerned.

This text is not specific to any particular National Health Service (NHS) ambulance trust or higher education institution. As the text is not specific to any one geographical location, you should expect to undertake further research for yourself on the areas that you are considering. Further research would be specific and focused on your chosen institution or institutions and ambulance NHS trust.

The text has chapters which are situated within specific parts; this is in direct response to students' comments about their studies. Students' comments can be categorised in four areas, which form the four parts of the text:

1   Preparation for becoming a student paramedic
2   Making the most of your academic study
3   Placement: preparing for and making the most of it
4   Transition to registration

The chapters within each part have been carefully selected to reflect the specific issues related to being a student paramedic on a higher education programme. The issues and subjects addressed in this text do not relate to any other subject area. The reader may wish to supplement the information discussed in this text with more generic study skills texts.

PART 1
Preparation for becoming a student paramedic

1 IS THIS THE RIGHT CAREER FOR ME?

A note about terminology

Some institutions use the word *programme* to explain the overall subject, other institutions use the word *course*. For example, the study of paramedic science may be called a programme or course. For ease of reading, the study of student paramedic will be referred to as a programme. The programme will be made up of building blocks that may be called modules, units or courses. This can be confusing. Our tip would be to make sure you understand the terminology, so you will understand how your programme of study will progress.

Some basics you need to be aware of

The title *paramedic* is a legally protected title; only professionals registered with the governing body, the Health and Care Professions Council (HCPC), are able to use the title of paramedic.

All higher education programmes that educate students to become paramedics have been through a stringent process of validation with the HCPC and adhere to their educational regulations and standards. Some higher education institutions (HEIs) have sought additional accreditation from the College of Paramedics, as the professional body for paramedics, and this will usually be visible in the institution's information about their paramedic programme.

All student paramedics are required to adhere to the *Standards of Conduct and Ethics for Students* (HCPC 2012a) throughout their period of study. Students need, as a requirement for public safety and protection, to be checked by the Disclosure and Barring Service. Instruction on the process will be provided by your university. This process identifies any criminal convictions and for some applicants will mean their application cannot proceed. A criminal conviction does not automatically preclude a candidate from applying to study for a paramedic qualification. However, it should be disclosed (as per statutory requirements) to the HEI which may discuss it with the partner placement provider(s) and make a decision on whether you would be suitable, depending on local policies. The candidate will also be screened by occupational health, in line with current Department of Health guidance. This will be organised by your university and/or your ambulance trust, if your programme of study involves employment by the ambulance service.

If successful in both academic and practical aspects of their studies, the student will exit the institution with the award and eligibility to apply for registration as a paramedic. Once registered, the paramedic must adhere to their employer's policies and procedures and demonstrate competence in the HCPC *Standards of Proficiency* for paramedics (2014) and abide by the HCPC *Standards of Conduct, Performance and Ethics* (2012a).

How is studying for a paramedic qualification different from other subjects?

There are several main differences that may (or may not) be applicable to the university programme you wish to apply to:

- You are receiving an academic and professional qualification; consequently, these types of programmes (mainly in health-care subjects) are longer than non-professionally regulated programmes. You will find that most programmes involve an academic year of 40–45 weeks.
- Some programmes involve employment with a National Health Service (NHS) ambulance trust, so you may not receive the university holidays as other students do.
- You may be required to undertake shift work whilst studying.
- The programme will cover a vast array of subjects that are relevant to the role. In addition, you will study specific clinical skills and associated anatomy and physiology.

⟲ Refer to Chapter 5 for more information on subjects covered.

Having provided a brief summary of how paramedic programmes differ from other programmes of study, the reality of being a student paramedic requires consideration.

Reality of the student paramedic role

The focus of this section is on giving student paramedics a voice, in order that you can read their advice based on reality, from their experience of the role of student paramedic. As individuals, students will view experiences differently, have different coping mechanisms and may have different motivations for studying for a paramedic qualification. The comments are from students in years 1, 2 and 3 of their studies (depending on the length of their programme). This is because the realities of the student paramedic role and your priorities do alter as time progresses throughout the programme of study.

Your programme will vary in the intensity with which it starts. Some programmes will begin quite slowly and flexibly, others will be *full on* for five days per week, with a copious amount of information being given at the beginning of the programme. One thing that most students have in common is that the learning environment will be different from what they are used to. Box 1.1 reflects that year 1 students generally wished they had undertaken some preparatory reading before starting their university studies. You may be surprised by the comments on the amount of university information and the change of lifestyle, as illustrated by the students' comments.

Box 1.1 Things year 1 students wished they had done to academically prepare for their studies

📖 I wish I had done more reading in things like anatomy and physiology before starting university, it is not my strong point and I feel left behind a little.

📖 Using the study skills and resources suggested by my university before starting my studies, I may have been quicker to get to grips with things like referencing and searching skills. I wasted a lot of time in the first few months.

📖 Our programme is unlike anything my friends are studying; they are studying academic subjects, like history. We were told this, but I don't think it is something I fully realised until I was in the midst of it.

📖 You are not told everything. Get used to reading, to top up what you are given in lectures.

> 📖 During the whole experience of the first nine months I felt like a fish out of water. I had forgotten a lot of my previous subject knowledge. Had I kept reading, even a little bit, during this time, I may have been more confident during lectures. Instead I am in a state of permanent catch-up and I don't like that feeling, it affects my confidence.

Box 1.1 highlights the fact that there are some strategies students can employ before they commence their university programme. Greater preparation before they commenced their programme of study may have made the transition into their academic studies easier. The preparation before the next year of study is equally as important, as described in Box 1.2.

As the comments in Box 1.2 highlight, some students in years 2 and 3 regret not making the most of their study periods or independent study time afforded to them in year 1. The comments relate to the change in academic level, the commitment required and the fact that as the student progresses it all seems to come together and makes more sense. Interestingly, the comments relating to simulation are both positive and negative.

From an academic and clinical perspective, simulation is something that you will need to practise. It is used extensively in both undergraduate and postgraduate studies and forms the basis of practical assessments within the academic environment. You may also find simulation being used by your mentors/PEds as an additional means of assessing your skills and knowledge when in practice. It can be an experience of personal growth as you respond to feedback given on your performance as you compare yourself to your colleagues, both in performance and knowledge. The student who tries to prepare for it is very sensible and probably the one who will get most from simulation experiences.

🔗 Refer to Chapter 6 for more information about learning in simulation.

Academic challenges are not the only concerns for students; finances seem to be a key theme for many. It can be difficult to manage your finances, involving juggling studies with paid employment. Sometimes students graduate with a debt to pay. Make sure you are fully informed before you embark on your studies (see Box 1.3), and make use of the student support available at your university.

Box 1.2 Comments from students in years 2/3 on preparing for the next academic year and academic study generally

📖 Read over your holiday time the things you are not happy with. I did not make the most of my study time in year 1 and I wish I had used it wisely. I have had to work hard to catch up.

📖 Year 1 was fun, but now it is getting more serious as we are being asked to do more in uni and in practice. More is expected of us and I don't want to look a fool, so I am working really hard. I wish I hadn't wasted so much of my time in year 1.

📖 As the modules/units pass it will make more sense, it all starts to come together and makes more sense in practice. You will have to work hard to be as good as you can be.

📖 A big jump in knowledge and learning, but in a good way.

📖 Study hard, you'll see the rewards.

📖 Go to the academic team if you are having any trouble, they will do all they can to help you or point you in the direction of someone who can.

📖 I hated simulation at the end of year 1, but now I prepare for it. I don't just go in there hoping for the best, I read up protocols, treatment and management and common medications. If I do my bit, then I get more from the days, rather than just being petrified. I learn so much more now. A previous student gave me this advice – thanks to them!

📖 Some people in my group hate learning in simulation, but I would rather make mistakes in this environment than on a real patient, when it could be really serious. It depends on your attitude, it isn't about the staff having a go at you, it is about you learning and making yourself a better student. Get over yourself.

📖 I really don't like my practice being scrutinised in a simulated environment, it is not real and does not reflect who I am when I am with real patients.

Box 1.3 Comments about the finances associated with paramedic study, from year 1 students

📖 Had I known how financially difficult it would be, I would have learnt how to save and budget better, before all my money had gone!

📖 Work, work, work and save, save, save, before you start your studies, otherwise you will be broke. Money disappears fast and that's without going out much, too.

📖 It is crazy, I want to focus on my studies, but I have now got two jobs to try and make ends meet. It is more difficult as time goes on too, as set hours for my extra jobs are impossible to juggle with shift work and increased academic demands.

📖 My friends on other paramedic programmes are worse and some are better off, I should have looked more closely at this before starting. I was just so desperate to start my career, but I may have got better results had I taken a year out to work and save.

As the comments in Box 1.3 from year 1 students highlight, finance needs to be given careful consideration. Finance is not the only factor in your decision-making process. As discussed in Chapter 2, there are many other important considerations when choosing a university programme.

🔗 Refer to Chapter 2 for more information about making your decisions.

Generally, all student paramedics cannot wait to have their first shift out in practice. The comments in Box 1.4 are generic and personal to each student and their own experiences, but they should give you an idea of the variety of feelings associated with the clinical environment. Be aware that programmes differ in the focus of placement. Some programmes will focus on the role and employment opportunities for the paramedic in other areas of the NHS, such as walk-in centres, general practitioner surgeries and emergency departments. Therefore, students may have less time on ambulance vehicles and more in wider NHS placement areas to prepare them for the reality of paramedics working outside the ambulance service role that is commonly expected by students. Programmes will reflect the diversity of the paramedic role in their particular locality and the partnerships developed between the institution, the NHS and ambulance service.

Box 1.4 Comments about the practice environment from year 1 students

📖 I did have some experience of dealing with/talking to people, but I could have done with having more.

📖 The distance I have to drive to and from placement is much more than I expected, it's expensive and we sometimes don't finish on time, so shifts are long.

📖 The job is quite physical, I wish I had worked on my basic strength before starting. It is difficult to eat well and healthily on shift and sometimes there is a lot of sitting about which doesn't help.

📖 It is not as busy on shift as I expected it to be.

📖 Shifts are great, but be prepared, sort your uniform out, get food ready, make sure you are on time and look smart and smile – that always helps, no one wants to see a miserable face. Oh, and learn to like tea!

📖 Be open-minded and get to know your mentor or PEd, you will learn so much if you are enthusiastic and want to learn.

📖 I have been a lot more involved than I expected and the majority of people are friendly and helpful. As in any job there are some people who do not get on. You have to be an adult and try to sort this out, or agree to disagree.

⌗ Refer to Chapters 8, 9 and 10 for more detail and explanation of the comments in Box 1.4.

The aim is that you will develop from being a student to become an educated professional, and the comments from year 2/3 students in Box 1.5 highlight aspects of this development. Not all students will achieve this progression and personal development over the course of their studies. However, it is the aim of paramedic higher education to produce graduates who employ critical thinking, are competent and skilled, and who provide high-quality care to their patients.

The development alluded to in Box 1.5 is made possible by commitment to academic study and learning in the clinical environment. This would be

---

Box 1.5 Year 2/3 students' comments about the practice environment

📖 I now keep an anonymised reflective journal of calls I go to that are quite out of the ordinary or are 'interesting' jobs, as they are things I am unlikely to see again. I don't have to, it is not something we have to do, but I learn better by reviewing things after they have happened and it helps me.

📖 Expectations of some ambulance staff who you thought were right in year 1, you now may begin to question, as you know more . . . think about how to manage this, it is a bit disappointing, but is the real world.

📖 Start attending at calls as early as you and your mentor or PEd feel is appropriate. The more experience you can get doing this now, the less of a shock it will be when you are registered.

📖 Use the knowledge and skills you get taught in uni, such as physical assessment, when you are with your mentor or PEd, otherwise you will forget them and this won't help your patient when you are the registered paramedic.

---

limited without a clear ability to manage your own time and an understanding of how you will progress towards achievements.

The comments made by year 1 students in Box 1.6 demonstrate some of their honest regrets related to their choices, in respect of study, career and placement issues. These students have embarked on the journey of beginning to understand themselves.

You will see from Box 1.6 that some of the aspects of being a student paramedic did indeed come as a shock. For some individuals it is not an easy transition into the role of being a university student or being a student paramedic. As the comments in Box 1.7 illustrate, the transition issues continue into the later study years.

Box 1.7 highlights the fact that the journey to knowing yourself continues long into your studies and probably long into the period after registration. We can also see that career choices shape some people's personalities over time. Some of the comments in Box 1.7 relate to self-awareness and the

Box 1.6 Comments from year 1 students about time and self-management

📖 Maybe I should have looked into becoming an ambulance support worker first, so I would have known more about what to expect, but I didn't want to wait until I was 21.

📖 I have struggled being away from home, it gets better, but had I known how tough it would be I may have stayed nearer home.

📖 I wasted too much time socialising and being one of my cohort, I have some major studying to do in the holidays. I fought hard for my place, I have let myself down by not maximising my potential, my results this year have been disappointing and it won't happen next year.

📖 I thought I was worldly wise – until I went into practice . . . it was not at all what I expected. Some awful and some great moments, I have learnt so so so much about myself and who I am. Maybe I could have been more use to patients had I known this before starting my studies.

📖 I have needed help to come to terms with some of the experiences I have had in practice, and my practice and academic team have been there for me. Stupidly, I thought by talking to them, it might affect my place on the programme – how wrong I was and I suffered on my own for too long before talking.

📖 I don't know what I expected, but this wasn't it.

concept of resilience. The following chapters will address in more detail the points made here.

The comments in Boxes 1.1–1.7 are *snippets* from a wide variety of students, and it is worth delving into these topics in more detail later in this text. Students' viewpoints will continue to be included throughout the chapters, to provide more detail in many areas and generally provide personal commentary.

Box 1.7 Year 2/3 students' comments relating to time and self-management

Our lecturer told us that over time we would change, I thought that was rubbish. How right she was, I meet up with my old friends now and think I have nothing in common with them. Actually I think they are immature and have no insight into the real world. Even though I play along at the time, when I am with them, the gaps between us meeting up are getting longer. I guess part of that is about who I am now and part of it is the career I have chosen.

Whether you like it or not this job will change your personality to an extent. This affects some people more than others.

One of my colleagues didn't like the people she was working with in practice, didn't like the [ambulance] service culture and found there was not enough time to care for people as she wanted. She left – it wasn't for her. It took a while to come to this conclusion, and was a brave move, I respect her for making the decision. I guess it is not for everyone.

If you are struggling in practice or uni – *talk* to someone and don't suffer in silence. It is not good or healthy to keep things to yourself.

If you are on a three-year programme, year 2 may be a bit of a grind, bear with it, work hard and use your study time wisely. Be disciplined with your time, it will pay off.

A more detailed comment on the reality of the student role

'I had been encouraged by people who knew me that I had the ability to handle the increasing levels of education the programme involved. In reality, as the programme progressed I had to give more and more time to study if I was to stay on target; this meant that the outside paid work, socialising and down time which had been possible during year 1 were increasingly squeezed in the subsequent years.

'A major help came in talking to students who were in the year ahead. They gave me pointers as to what was coming which meant I spent some of the holidays reading up on subjects we would study when we returned to uni. This proved invaluable as I would have struggled to keep up without it.

'As far as placement experience went I had little idea what to expect. I knew it wasn't going to be like the popular hospital dramas on TV but also, unlike other students, I had not come from a St John/British Red Cross background so had limited ambulance experience. In some ways this may have helped in that I had no preconceived ideas about how things should be done and this caused me to ask lots of questions and learn things from scratch.'

The more detailed response above has been included to enable the reader to understand some of the points considered and strategies used by one student before and during their paramedic studies. Having an awareness of the potential issues you may encounter may help you prepare and plan for your future studies. The comments presented here do not just reflect the good parts about being a student paramedic, they provide a realistic picture.

The detail provided in the following chapters should help you develop a more detailed understanding of the student paramedic role and the idiosyncrasies of studying for a paramedic qualification. However, it would be unwise to only examine the student perspective; the academic, mentor and PEd viewpoints will enable you to appreciate a wider perspective than that of the student.

The responses in Box 1.8 are from academics and paramedic mentors/PEds in response to the question 'what makes a student paramedic successful?'

Gaining 'appropriate' experience

Appropriate is a term that students report is widely used by staff at HEIs. It is an ambiguous term, and what one academic means by it could be different from what is meant by another. Box 1.9 presents some interpretations of the term.

What is 'appropriate' experience?

The term *appropriate* can encompass many experiences. One of the most important skills to acquire through experience is being able to communicate with a stranger. It is possible to improve your communication skills,

Box 1.8 What makes a student paramedic successful?

Paramedic mentor/PEd response: The most successful students I have mentored have been those that cared about their patients. Students can be taught academic and clinical skills but we can't teach them caring, empathy, common sense or life experience. If a student has these raw materials to begin with the rest invariably follows. These qualities together with a sense of humour, a pride in the profession and a willingness to learn will ensure success in both placement and university.

Academic responses: The ethos of higher education is often somewhat of a shock to students. You are 'treated like a grown-up' and are expected to take a great deal of responsibility for your own learning. There is limited time in class in which to teach you, and modules specify a large number of hours you will need to commit to your own study. Pre-reading is invaluable and students that have taken time to increase their knowledge before the programme will be at an advantage. You don't need a specific reading list for this, generic anatomy and physiology textbooks are a good place to start.

Your module guides are the most valuable documents you will receive on your programme, as they highlight the content, learning outcomes and assessment criteria of the modules and help you to study effectively.

Do not stay silent if you feel you are struggling or falling behind. Academic teams and mentors are there to help and will go out of their way to support you.

Paramedic/PEd response: I believe the key to being a successful student paramedic is to embrace your chosen career pathway and academic journey with true wholehearted commitment and dedication, with a passion to achieve your goal and with an informed and detailed understanding of the programme in which you will study. Being open and prepared to accept anything offered to you throughout your study enables you to build both varied and fulfilling experiences. Additionally, self-control is vital in order to manage time effectively in order to complete academic assignments whilst also attending shift working placements and remembering to live a 'professional' student life, all of which is slightly different from students on other non-professional/clinical academic programmes.

Box 1.9 Interpretations of the word 'appropriate', in respect of gaining appropriate experience

🎓 **Academic response:** In academic terms and particularly when talking about prior 'appropriate' experience, this is taken to mean 'suitable'. Just because your prior experience may not be of a medical nature, that does not mean it is not appropriate and will not be valuable to your role as a paramedic. Students who have some experience of life tend to fare better in caring and health professions. In this context, then, the life experience of the student would be deemed appropriate if this can be communicated in an application form or at interview. The important thing is that you can recognise how the knowledge, skills and attributes that you have developed through prior experience can be transferable to the role of paramedic.

🚨 **Paramedic mentor/PEd response:** The term 'appropriate', particularly in placement, is often used in the context of behaviour. Ask yourself: is something suitable in the circumstances? This can apply to any number of things from humour, dress, the way in which you communicate with your patients or how you behave towards your colleagues.

🚨 **Paramedic mentor/PEd response:** The term 'appropriate' refers to transferable and learned behaviours, actions, attitudes and knowledge acquired from health-care environments, where patient, relative, and staff interactions occur.

📖 **Student paramedic response**: 'Appropriate' means having or doing something which brings a positive outcome or advantage to you or a situation.

and indeed it will be essential to become more aware of the ways in which you can do so. Having experience of talking and establishing a rapport with strangers is a great starting point.

Any participative role where you communicate with strangers on a regular basis will be valuable. This could include working in a shop, volunteer work, or working with vulnerable members of the community on a voluntary/paid basis, such as a residential care home. There are many more, as can be seen by the student comment below.

> **Student paramedic comment:** Obviously paramedic practice involves caring for people in a pre-hospital setting . . . however, so much of this involves non-clinical aspects such as communication, empathy, listening skills and decision-making. Though I gained some experience of basic health care working with disabled pupils, in my previous job as a special needs teaching assistant, I learnt just as much about effective communication, persuasiveness and conflict resolution through working with the able-bodied children who were also pupils at the school.
>
> Appropriate experience is not just knowing how to put someone's arm in a sling, it's as much about learning how to listen, talk, reassure and bring calm to people . . . and you don't need to get a Saturday job in a hospital to develop these things, you can develop your 'people skills' just as much working in a retail environment as in a clinical one.

The practical skills that a paramedic needs to possess will be taught to you throughout your programme. In many respects, this is the easy part, the more complex part is most definitely fine-tuning and excelling at communication in all its forms (see the suggested reading at the end of this chapter).

🕮 Refer to Chapter 9 for more information on communication.

Transferable skills

At university open days, lecturers and paramedic lecturer practitioners/ associate lecturers are often asked what experience candidates need before applying. This is not an easy question to answer and to some extent is subjective. Each candidate is unique and as such will have varied experiences. The easiest way to answer this question is to think about *transferable skills*. What attributes, skills and personality traits do you possess that you think will be required for your chosen career (see the reflection point below)? Whilst some candidates will have direct experience with patients and providing patient care, others may not, and this is not necessarily a negative – for instance, see the student comments in Boxes 1.4 and 1.5. Think about the career you are considering. It is fundamentally about communicating with and caring for people of all ages. So if you have any experience working with people (as an employee or on a voluntary basis) it could be considered appropriate.

It is also important that you consider your own personal qualities and compare these to those you believe a paramedic should possess. Self-awareness is also an important part of being able to help others. Being in tune with yourself may enable you to be more astute and responsive to others' needs.

> **Reflection: points to consider**
>
> Clarify for yourself what you think the role of a paramedic is. Make a list of your answers.
>
> What personal attributes would you say are valuable?
>
> Think about any voluntary or paid work you have done. What personal attributes are transferable to the paramedic role as you described it above?

Communication is essential and is one of the six Cs of the NHS rolled out in December 2012 as part of the Compassion in Practice national nursing strategy. Communication is consistently discussed in the government's response to the Francis Report (Department of Health 2013b) as requiring improvement, and should hold a central role in any education of health-care professionals. As Stevenson (2014) reports, many other health professions, in addition to nursing, are also adopting the six Cs approach. Therefore communication skills will be discussed as part of your studies, but it is worth noting these skills generally take time to develop, hone and practise. A caring nature cannot be taught. Of course patients are best placed to distinguish if a health-care professional cares or not. Many programmes involve users/carers in the teaching and assessment of students to help to develop communication skills in a safe environment.

The NHS is under constant scrutiny from politicians and the media. Since 2010 attention has been focused on issues with the quality of care and the professionals who provide the care (Department of Health 2013a, 2013b). Whilst the cases highlighted to date are predominantly hospital-based, the changes and focus for all NHS trusts highlighted in the Francis Report (Department of Health 2013a) equally apply to NHS ambulance trusts and employees. This level of scrutiny is something you need to be aware of. Communication is at the heart of the NHS and is a crucial element of patient care. Gaining experience in an environment where you need to communicate with people is, therefore, extremely valuable.

& Refer to Chapter 9 for current issues in health care and more information on the six Cs.

Why is gaining experience important?

Generally, patients do not call for ambulance assistance lightly; it is a conscious decision that is for many patients a last resort. Many patients you will see are frightened, anxious and unwell. Your ability to communicate effectively with them will help to put them at their ease, reduce their anxiety, instil confidence in your ability to help them and make their overall experience as positive as possible (Street 2012). But handling patients badly can have long-lasting consequences for patients and their carers.

Shouldn't I be getting experience with the ambulance service?

Due to health and safety issues and ambulance trust policy, it is extremely difficult to obtain experience observing on ambulance vehicles. But although you may not be able to gain prior experience, it may benefit you to speak to people who are paramedics, ask about their study and how they progressed to the role of paramedic. Ask what they do during the course of a shift: this should provide a realistic picture – more realistic than the media portrays. Find out if your region employs paramedics in areas other than the ambulance service. You may be able to observe their working practices and discuss with them how this differs from the role of the paramedic working for an ambulance service.

Television documentaries usually focus on the ambulance service paramedic and are heavily edited, as their role is primarily to entertain the viewer. What you will see in documentaries are snippets of care episodes that are usually not realistic in terms of the amount of time you spend with patients; they mostly include footage of dramatic patient interactions/incidents and are not a true reflection of what happens during the course of a shift. Speak to student paramedics and paramedic lecturers when you visit university open events. Visit the College of Paramedics website, and read the section about ambulance trusts and frequently asked questions. You may also find the reading list at the end of this chapter useful.

Doing this research yourself should help you prepare for the programme and also be ready with questions that are focused and specific to the university you wish to apply to.

Is there competition for a place to study for a paramedic qualification?

The short answer to this question is yes. Competition is fierce, but there are more HEIs commissioned to run paramedic programmes now than there were a few years ago, so this may change over time.

> **Student paramedic comment:** I did not have the option of joining the ambulance service patient transport and working my way up to becoming a paramedic as this route was no longer available in my area. So if I wanted to become a paramedic the direct entry route via university was the only way. I had been warned that competition was fierce to get a place at university, with over 700 people applying for the 20 available places in the year I began. Fortunately I got a place!
>
> I remember on the first day 20 of us sat in a circle in a classroom. Our programme leader told us that approximately 35 other people had applied to sit in each of the chairs we now occupied, yet we had been given the opportunity. He told us to 'look after our place' as it had already been hard won. This really motivated me to do my best, I didn't want to squander the place that someone else didn't get the chance to have.

Popularity

The role of paramedic is very popular as a choice for career. It is a dynamic, multi-functional role within the NHS and one which can be developed into a career path for paramedics much more so now than ever before. The career choices for individuals once registered as a paramedic are numerous and personal development is expected. These opportunities lead to paramedics going to work overseas, working with general practitioners, in walk-in centres, in emergency departments or in research or education. Much more than ever before, paramedics can choose to focus their career in a way that evolves to suit their interests and expertise and ultimately benefits patient care.

The interview process

The purpose of this section is to give an overview of what may happen at interview. This information is deliberately quite generic and more detail would be provided by the institution that is inviting you to interview. All HEIs will interview prospective candidates across the academic year before the programme begins. Candidates will usually be sent details of the type of interview process the university uses. Some HEIs use face-to-face panel interviews (with university and/or ambulance trust staff), others use mini multiple interviews (MMIs). MMIs involve candidates rotating around a series of simulation stations and being asked questions by a number of different interviewers. The HEI will usually provide details as required.

> **Student paramedic comment:** Like everyone I prepared for my uni interviews by trying to second-guess what the interviewers would want to know and swotting in those areas. I probably had a load of rehearsed answers which tried to show that even my hobbies had some element of 'transferable skill' to being a paramedic. I went to four interviews and got two offers. I think now that the offers I got came out of those interviews where I got away from my 'prepared speeches' and was able to show something of who I actually am whilst talking to the interviewers. 'Knowing your stuff' is obviously important, but 'being yourself' is just as important – interviewers want to see who you are not just what you know.

The standard process for many HEIs is for candidates to also sit a short mathematics and English paper in addition to the interview. Some HEIs and partner ambulance trusts also require candidates to pass a fitness test, and this may take place before or after interview. There may be additional requirements that are specific to the institution; again details/guidance would be given to candidates before interview.

What to do if I am not successful?

Although it may seem like the end of the world, it may not be the end of your journey. With the popularity of paramedic education, it is not surprising that many candidates are unsuccessful on the first occasion. From experience, one common reason is that interviewees are unable to clearly articulate that they know what paramedics actually do. If you still wish to pursue this career choice, try to obtain some feedback on why you were not successful. Bear in mind that due to the vast numbers of candidates, many universities are not able to resource staff to provide dedicated, personalised feedback. If you gain this information, reflect on what you have been told, across the course of the year.

If you are not able to gain this information:

● Review your personal statement.
● Be realistic about your previous experiences (voluntary and employed).
● Reflect on the experiences other people had whom you met at interview.
● Perhaps think about widening your experience.

You may want to consider if this is what you really want, and how much you are prepared to commit to attaining a place. Review your supporting statement and update it, in line with your added year of experience(s) before reapplying to UCAS.

Use your time constructively. Think about what other candidates may have had (in terms of experience) that you may not have; paid care work experience is always a good option if possible. You may find other doors open for you and find something you unexpectedly enjoy doing – who knows? If not, you will still be developing and practising your communication and care skills during this time.

The positive is that, should you reapply, you will know what to expect from the interview process!

Suggested reading

Bach, S. and Grant, A. (2009) *Communication and Interpersonal Skills for Nurses*. Exeter: Learning Matters.

(Whilst the title of this text includes another professional group, much of the communication theory discussed in the text is transferable to the role of paramedic.)

Blaber, A.Y. (ed.) (2012) *Foundations for Paramedic Practice: A Theoretical Perspective* (2nd edn). Maidenhead: Open University Press.

College of Paramedics (2013) Paramedic higher education information programmes. Available at: https://www.collegeofparamedics.co.uk/downloads/Paramedic_Higher_Education.pdf (accessed 18 January 15).

College of Paramedics website: https://www.collegeofparamedics.co.uk/ (accessed 18 January 2015)

Department of Health (2013a) *Report of the Mid Staffordshire NHS Foundation Trust Public Inquiry: Executive Summary.* London: The Stationery Office.

Department of Health (2013b) *Patients First and Foremost: The Government's Initial Responses to the Francis Inquiry.* London: The Stationery Office.

Health and Care Professions Council (2012a) *Standards of Conduct, Performance and Ethics.* London: HCPC. Available at: http://www.hcpc-uk.org/assets/documents/10003B6EStandardsofconduct,performanceandethics.pdf (accessed 18 January 2015).

Health and Care Professions Council (2012b) *Guidance on Conduct and Ethics for Students.* London: HCPC. Available at: http://www.hcpc-uk.org/assets/documents/10002C16Guidanceonconductandethicsforstudents.pdf (accessed 18 January 2015).

Health and Care Professions Council (2014) *Standards of Proficiency. Paramedics.* London: HCPC. Available at: http://www.hpc-uk.org/assets/documents/1000051CStandards_of_Proficiency_Paramedics.pdf (accessed 18 January 2015).

NHS Careers: Paramedic. Available at: http://www.nhscareers.nhs.uk/explore-by-career/ambulance-service-team/careers-in-the-ambulance-service/paramedic/ (accessed 18 January 2015).

Stevenson, J. (2014) NHS England to rollout '6Cs' nursing values to all health care service staff. *Nursing Times*, 23 April. Available at: http://www.nursingtimes.net/nursing-practice/specialisms/management/exclusive–6cs-nursing-values-to-be-rolled-out-to-all-nhs-staff/5070102.article (accessed 18 January 2015).

Street, P.A. (2012) Interpersonal communication: a foundation of practice. In A.Y. Blaber (ed.) *Foundations for Paramedic Practice: A Theoretical Perspective* (2nd edn). Maidenhead: Open University Press.

2 CHOOSING A PROGRAMME AND UNIVERSITY

Do your research. This is an important decision.
The main route to becoming a Health and Care Professions Council (HCPC) registered paramedic in England is via a programme at a higher education institution (HEI). There are others, such as via the Open University (where you need to be an employee of an ambulance trust and have placement time supported by your employer), but the focus of this book will be on the higher education route, where HEIs work in partnership with their local NHS ambulance trust. It has not always been this way.

Prior to the development of higher education (HE) programmes, many paramedics started their careers being employed by an ambulance service and working on patient transport vehicles (for this you had to be at least 21 years of age). Then they would undertake ambulance service or in-house training to become technician grade staff, and then additional training to become a registered paramedic.

Many paramedics have gone on to combine working and studying to achieve certificates, diplomas, degrees, master's degrees and PhDs. Some clinical staff have years of practical clinical experience and a variety of academic qualifications, and will act as mentors or paramedic educators (PEds) for student paramedics. Additionally, many staff act as mentors/PEds after completing a short mentorship/PEd module, and sometimes this forms the start of their journey to post-registration studies, though sometimes individuals wish to complete the mentorship/PEd module and do not wish to undertake further academic study.

In the NHS it is very much up to the individual clinician how they choose to develop themselves and how their continuing professional development (CPD) will be used, and the focus of their CPD will often depend on their interests.

Level of study

Undergraduate HE programmes can take the form of certificates, diplomas, foundation degrees or degrees. Knowing the differences is an important part of your decision-making (see Table 2.1).

∂ Refer to Chapter 3 for more information on level of study.

Table 2.1 Various levels of undergraduate study

Undergraduate year	Academic level of study	Certificate	Diploma	Foundation degree	Degree
1	4	✓	✓	✓	✓
2	5		✓	✓	✓
3	6				✓

As Table 2.1 shows, the academic level is indicative of the qualification obtained after the programme of study. The variety of titles given to the programmes indicates the academic level of study achieved. One of the most common misconceptions is the title *degree*. The government coined the phrase 'foundation degrees' during their inception in the 1990s. Generally foundation degrees (FDs) are of 2 years' duration and students complete academic levels 4 and 5 only. The subjects studied for the paramedic specialism will be broadly similar, but some FDs will not include research in much (if any) depth. Bachelor of Science (BSc) or Bachelor of Arts (BA) degrees will include a research component and generally a lengthy piece of research-focused work called a *dissertation*.

When distinguishing between BSc and BSc(Hons) programmes, the 'Hons' part of the award may or may not be linked to the dissertation. For example, in some institutions students can exit the institution with a BSc if they fail to submit/choose not to complete their dissertation. In other institutions the dissertation is part of the overall award and failure to complete the dissertation will mean the student cannot be awarded their degree at all. This is not usual. To be clear, with all pieces of work, students are generally allowed a second and possibly a third attempt, should they fail (or refer) at the first attempt.

There are many reasons why people choose programmes at different academic levels. These reasons may not always be so obvious and in many cases are personal; see Case Studies 2.1 and 2.2.

CASE STUDY 2.1

Tim has a BSc(Hons) in Sports Science and as a result has a substantial student loan. He is reluctant to accumulate more debt and has therefore chosen to apply for diploma-level study over 2 years, rather than a three-year BSc(Hons). Whilst Tim is capable of studying at level 6 (as his success in sports science proves), the financial situation is a major consideration for him.

Tim in Case Study 2.1 should be pursuing BSc level study, but the financial anomalies and difficulties are substantial enough to affect his decision-making. As Case Study 2.2 highlights, sometimes candidates apply to university courses without considering the potential issues they may face.

CASE STUDY 2.2

Sally is considering applying for university paramedic study. Sally has a strong support network with her friends and family. She is finding her access course hard work but wants to be a paramedic. Sally does not want to move away from home, she wants to study nearby. The only programmes offered at universities near to Sally's home are at BSc level, so she is only applying to these universities. In conversations with her friends and family, Sally says she may find study at BSc level too challenging, but is applying anyway.

Sally may not gain entry to a BSc programme. If she is struggling with her access course, she may not meet the entry criteria for BSc study, as generally this will be higher than for foundation degree or diploma-level study. Case Studies 2.1 and 2.2 help to explain that sometimes students apply for and end up on programmes for a variety of reasons. Decision-making is not straightforward or without external influences. This misunderstanding around levels of study, together with the complex financial situation surrounding paramedic study, can lead to extremely varied educational standards of students within a cohort of student paramedics. Hopefully the case studies have highlighted that each student has their own personal circumstances, competing demands and situations to take into account when choosing their level of study.

One important consideration is that the current recommendation by the College of Paramedics is that all registrant paramedics hold level 5 qualifications by 2015 in order to register with the HCPC, followed by level 6 by 2019. This recommendation to raise the academic threshold and subsequent entry to the HCPC register comes from the findings of the Paramedic Evidence-based Education Project (Lovegrove 2013; College of Paramedics 2014). The College of Paramedics (2014) makes a distinction between the regions of the UK, stating that entry to the register should be at academic level 6 in England, Wales and Northern Ireland and SHE level 3 (SCQF9) in Scotland by academic year 2015/16, with all regions continuing to work towards the 2019 target as far as is practicable. It has been recognised that raising the academic threshold is best for the future of the paramedic profession and ultimately better for patient care.

Location – near home or further away?

Again this is a personal decision. Some students will be restricted by their personal circumstances and what HEIs near them offer in terms of provision and academic level of paramedic education. Other students will want to move away from their family and friends and want to experience university life.

Increasingly, students are choosing to live nearer to where they call home (whether that be near friends/family or not) and attend the nearest paramedic programme to them. They are, however, generally not living with their parent(s), choosing to stay close to home but living independently. There may be many reasons for this but support networks, student fees and subsequent debt on leaving university are certainly considerations for many students (Grove 2014).

Student paramedic comment: Deciding whether to live away or stay closer to home for university is a big decision. For some, they love the freedom it gives them and opportunities associated with this. For me, this has not been the case. Many factors can influence reasons why you may struggle being away from where you call home. I am a mature student and this is my second time at university. I was used to working full-time, having my own place, money to spend and being able to see friends and family. It has been a big shock returning to being a student, living with strangers and surviving off little money.

Student paramedic comment: Studying away from home for me was a certainty as none of the local universities provided a paramedic degree and the degree was what I wanted. So it was more of a case of how far I was willing to go. For me, moving away was part of growing up and becoming independent, ready for having a full-time job at the end of the programme, but the distance from home was still a worry. Looking back, the distance in miles was less of a problem than I thought, and only makes a difference when travelling home for holidays.

The programme itself and placements are exciting but can be strenuous enough without moving house and meeting new friends and work colleagues. Sometimes it has been slightly challenging being so far away from the normality of home, but a strong circle of close friends and help from university tutors have proved invaluable when I needed them, and overall it has been an easy transition. I would recommend anyone thinking of moving away to give some thought to moving first, but it is more than possible and for me it was a great decision.

The comments above provide insight into some of the factors influential in decision-making for two students. As they demonstrate, support networks are an important consideration.

Support networks

Think about who provides you with support when you need it. Do you think you can manage with these important people being quite a distance away, or would you prefer to keep them nearby? Any health-care role involves personal investment in your patients and clients. This can be extremely rewarding, but not always a happy experience and without distress for the patient, their family and perhaps yourself. You may need the support of your established network, in addition to the new friends you will be making and the colleagues and staff you will get to know as your studies progress.

∂ Refer to Chapter 13 for more on support and resilience.

As you can see from the students comments below, support networks are extremely important to student paramedics, in whatever guise.

Student paramedic comment: I had a good support network in my family (being married, with a grown-up son) who were always encouraging of what I was doing. I found, though, that as my clinical experience developed and the number of 'difficult' call-outs I went to increased I became more and more selective about what I would tell my family. This was partly as I did not want to upset them with some of the things I'd seen, but also because as you progress in your paramedic experience you realise that relatives and friends can't always understand or appreciate some aspects of the job – you have to be in it to fully understand it. As a result you keep some things to yourself. This can be difficult in terms of ensuring you don't let things get on top of you, especially if you've been to a traumatic call-out where you encountered something upsetting. That's where I began to rely more and more on my fellow student paramedics (who were also encountering some things for the first time). We were a very close knit cohort and strongly supported each other. Also my paramedic mentor and programme tutors were brilliant in supporting me/us. I guess you develop different levels of support from different people as you progress through the programme. It ties in a lot with developing your personal resilience.

Student paramedic comment: Losing my support network has had a big impact on deciding whether living so far from friends and family is worth it. Travelling back home every month or so takes a big toll on you not only financially but also physically, which can make keeping up with studies and placements hard work.

Student paramedic comment: A support network is important whilst on a programme like this, as it can be quite intense and emotionally challenging at times. I am quite a distance from home and it is impossible to keep travelling home. Of course I keep in contact, but need to become independent too. My advice would be to make sure you find someone who you are comfortable talking to, and don't be afraid to ask for help or support from university, they've dealt with it all before and really do help. Good luck!

As mentioned by the students in the comments above, support networks come in all shapes and sizes, and each student will have an individual approach to establishing and maintaining these networks. It is important not to overlook the importance and value of thinking about your existing support networks and being realistic about your individual requirements.

Reflection: points to consider

Having read the comments from students about the importance of choosing a university, the 'home or away' decision and the importance of your support networks, write a list of the pros and cons of your university choices. This may help you think more deeply and may highlight issues that you had not previously considered.

Visiting the universities

Visit the Universities and Colleges Admissions Service website for a list of programmes offered and then explore the specific university websites that are relevant to your choices. Also visit the College of Paramedics website for information pertaining to students.

Think about your current studies and what level of study best suits you. Do internet research about the various programmes on offer and make a shortlist of HEIs that you wish to consider. Look at the wider website for the HEI and look at things that are important to you, such as sports facilities, social clubs, or student events. Although programmes are competitive, it is really important that you will be happy during your period of study in an institution.

Attend open days where at all possible. Here you usually have the opportunity to hear from the lecturers running the programmes and the current students, and you can ask questions that may be generic or specific to the programme. You will get a sense of the academic environment, location and whether the programme is what you expected or not, as the student comment below illustrates.

Student paramedic comment: Open days are a must. You get a better feel for a place by going there than by just reading a prospectus. You also meet fellow 'wannabe' paramedic students who you keep bumping into at different uni open days! This is especially good if some of you make it to the same cohort at the same uni – meaning you already have a couple of friends on the first day!

The chance to talk to the programme leaders/current students/past students is often part of the open day experience. At my university we got the chance to speak to current students on their own without the tutors. This meant we could ask whatever we liked and get a true idea of what the programme involved. I thought this was a very good idea and made me want to attend this uni more than the others I'd seen.

Let's talk about money

Embarking on a university programme is a big decision and one really important factor to consider is the financial commitment.

Fee status of the programme

University programme fees are something you need to research for yourself. At the time of writing, the picture is extremely varied across England for paramedic programmes. The same cannot be said of other health professional courses. For example, student nurses do not pay tuition fees (these are paid by the NHS) and they receive a bursary (amount variable, depending on personal circumstances). This is not the case with paramedic education, although the professional body, the College of Paramedics, has made representations to the Department of Health to address the anomalies. As you can see from the examples in Table 2.2, the situation is hugely variable and you need to establish the situation at each university and their partner ambulance trust to whom you wish to apply.

Table 2.2 Examples of the potential variation in fee status

Student	University fees	Any funding provided to the student by the local clinical commissioning group (CCG)	Travel expenses	Uniform
1	£9000	None	None	Not provided
2	£9000	None	Paid	Provided
3	£9000	Monthly amount paid direct to student	Paid	Provided
4	Paid by CCG to university	None	None	Provided
5	Paid by CCG to university	Monthly amount paid direct to student	Paid	Provided

As you will notice, student 5 in Table 2.2 is financially better off than student 1. Unfortunately these financial irregularities are a reality and may well affect your decision-making. These differences are something that you need to be aware of and should be explored during your research and visits to the universities. In addition to the programme costs, you will need to factor in the cost of living for your chosen location of study.

Accommodation costs

At the risk of stating the obvious, parts of England vary considerably in terms of the cost of accommodation and the cost of living – rent, buying food and socialising. Research this carefully and be realistic. You will need time away from your studies to relax, so try to factor this in.

Travel costs

As with other health-care professions, paramedic programmes will involve working with paramedics on ambulances and other vehicles. You will need to get to your placement area. Research the areas that you may be expected to travel to for clinical placement, and look at the worst-case scenario in terms of distances that you may need to travel. Also consider how often you are expected to do this and over how long a period, as the costs involved will add up over time.

> **Student paramedic comment:** I would say you definitely need your own car. You can use public transport for a lot of things, but if you finish a shift after an overrun at 2a.m. you'll be waiting a long time at the bus stop (possibly in the freezing rain!). I can't think of a student in our cohort who didn't have their own transport – it's a necessity.

How will you get to the clinical placement: using your own car or by public transport? When considering shifts, it may not be possible to get public transport to some areas, or after the end of shifts. Your own personal safety is also a huge consideration – you may be finishing a shift in the early hours and need to get home safely.

Ask about reimbursement of travel costs. As with funding, some programmes may offer this, some may not. If travel costs are reimbursed, be realistic that you will have to pay for the travel up front and then claim costs back. There will be a delay in your receiving the money you have already paid out.

Working while studying

Ideally, your studies should be a priority so that you can achieve your potential. However, HEIs are mindful of the financial situations of their students and understand that many students need to supplement their income by undertaking paid work throughout the duration of their studies. Many HEIs will provide guidance on this with regard to an appropriate balance between paid work and study. In discussion with colleagues in other universities, they usually recommend no more than 15–20 hours of paid work per week. However, this will not be suitable for all students, as the student comment below indicates.

Student paramedic comment: Managing your money through your studies is something you definitely need to keep on top of if you don't want to find yourself struggling more than a student normally has to struggle. I would say it is possible to have a job outside of study in the first year; however, in the second (and if you have a third year) it becomes increasingly difficult. It's not impossible, I know other students managed it but I couldn't have. I saved as much money as I could prior to starting my studies and worked hard to earn money beforehand so that I didn't have to get a paying job during the programme and could concentrate on my studies. I've still come out with a student debt, but at least it's not as big as students who had to pay fees on top of living costs.

You will come out with a student debt, it's unavoidable. However, just how big that debt is can be up to you in your choice of uni, your financial preparation before starting, and in how closely you manage your money during the programme.

As a student on a paramedic programme, you are likely to be expected to undertake some shift work. If you have never worked shifts previously, you may find your sleep becomes disturbed and you struggle to balance shifts on placement with study and outside work commitments. You also need to consider what type of paid work may fit into your programme, as the student's comment above highlights. For instance, if you have regular work each Saturday, is it possible to keep your Saturday job if you have to undertake placement hours on some Saturdays? This is another aspect to consider carefully.

& Refer to Chapter 8 and the section on shift work for more detail

Can you afford it?

Unfortunately, the reality of the situation is that a lack of money may impact upon your studies. It is therefore really important that you take into consideration all of the points raised in this chapter. It may be that you postpone your decision to study for a year, whilst you gather some health-care experience and accumulate some funds, so you can solely concentrate on your programme. This is not the end of the world. Be realistic about the demands of the study, placement, shifts, and potential lack of money, and make your decision accordingly. At least you know what you are letting yourself in for! Unfortunately, the drain on finances is not just related to your accommodation and living expenses – there is potentially driving instruction to consider.

To drive or not to drive?

The picture is varied in respect of driving. The reasons why this is the case require some explanation. Currently there is no requirement to hold a full UK manual driving licence to register with the HCPC as a paramedic (HCPC 2014).

Yes, there are other paramedic roles that do not involve driving, such as cyclist paramedics and paramedics working on oil rigs. Other than the ambulance service, the more usual paramedic roles are working in primary care in GP surgeries and walk-in centres, and sometimes in EDs. However, the more unusual posts (cyclist, oil rig paramedics) usually require experience as a paramedic in order to be shortlisted for interview. So at some point, if you want to work for an ambulance service, you will need to hold a full manual UK driving licence. However, there are restrictions on people driving emergency vehicles with certain medical conditions (see DVLA 2013).

The picture is further muddled by what is known as category C1. The weight of ambulances becomes an issue here; generally they weigh in excess of 3500 kilograms. After 1997, changes outlined by the DVLA (see https://www.gov.uk/old-driving-licence-categories) meant that passing a full UK manual test no longer entitled you to drive vehicles in excess of 3500 kg, as it had previously.

Many applicants to paramedic programmes will also need to take an additional theory and practical test to have category C1 on their existing full UK manual driving licence. The point at which students are required/need to do this will depend on the programme of study and their age. Some programmes involve part employment with ambulance trusts, therefore for these programmes students need to have C1 on their licence before starting their studies. Other programmes require just the full manual UK driving licence and, if you do not have C1 category, it may be suggested that you plan this into your vacation periods so you possess it before completion. Others do not require you to be able to drive, such is the variation.

There is a financial implication to obtaining this category, so you should enquire about the costs involved from driving schools with experience of preparing student paramedics for the C1 tests. Other programmes may not require you to drive at all, but be mindful of the issues of getting to and from your clinical placements, as detailed in the previous section. See Table 2.3 for further details on the process.

Table 2.3 Details of C1 driving category and blue-light driving course

Process for obtaining category C1 on your driving licence

- Once you have passed and are in receipt of your full UK manual driving licence you are eligible to apply for your provisional C1 licence (you need to be over 18 years of age).
- To apply for your provisional C1 obtain the following forms (online or from a main post office):
  - o D2 (application) and
  - o D4 (medical).
- Before submitting the forms for provisional C1 a medical is required.
- Contact your GP, enquire about cost. Each GP will have a scale of charges.
- Once the medical is completed, submit both forms.
- Once you have received your provisional C1 licence you can book the Driving Theory and Hazard Perception Test (telephone 0300 2001122 (option 1) or online at http://www.direct.gov.uk/en/Motoring/Motoringtransactions/DG_066356).
- There are some specific books that may be recommended by your driving school, specific to the C1 theory and driving test. As a starting point, the official Highway Code is available online at the above web link.
- Contact a C1 driving provider to book the practical lessons and part of the test.

IHCD blue-light driving course

- You will need to have held your full UK manual driving licence for 1 year before you can start the IHCD blue light driving course.
- Your university and ambulance trust will be able to provide more details once you reach this stage.
- This will be required at different stages, depending on your institution's arrangements with the ambulance trust. For example, some programmes will not include blue light driving – it will be undertaken as part of your induction when you obtain a job as a paramedic with an ambulance trust. Other programmes arrange it with the partner ambulance trust, as part of your programme.

> **Student paramedic comment:** You are going to need a C1 on your driving licence if you didn't pass your test before 1997. The cost of getting this is significant, so you need to factor it in. Even if you already have a C1 category on your licence (as I did) it's worth getting a couple of lessons in an ambulance equivalent vehicle if you've not driven one before, just so you know what it's like. You don't want the first time you get behind the wheel of something bigger than a car to be on the first day of your blue-light driving course.

Once you possess category C1 on your driving licence you will need to complete an Institute of Health and Care Development (IHCD) *blue-light* driving course. This is usually managed by the partner ambulance trust or the paramedic's first employer (if they choose employment by an ambulance trust); see Table 2.3 for more detail.

However, it is likely that most registrants' first employed post as a paramedic will be with an NHS ambulance trust, mostly working on an ambulance, perhaps occasionally on a solo responder vehicle. Therefore, it is commonplace for NHS ambulance trusts to stipulate that applicants also have category C1 on their full manual UK driving licence. Some universities may have a partnership approach to this issue with their local NHS ambulance trust, such as the trust lending students the money for the C1 tests and the student paying this back once they are employed.

This chapter has addressed many aspects that require the applicant to be self-aware, realistically address the potential difficulties and be honest about the realities of undertaking a paramedic programme. Next we will consider how to make the most of studying the academic study portion of a paramedic programme.

Suggested reading and websites

College of Paramedics (2014) *Paramedic Curriculum Guidance* (3rd edn). Bridgwater: College of Paramedics. Available at: https://www.collegeofparamedics.co.uk/downloads/Curriculum_Guidance_2014.pdf (accessed 18 February 2015).

DVLA (2013) *Current Medical Guidelines: DVLA Guidance for Professionals*. Available at: https://www.gov.uk/current-medical-guidelines-dvla-guidance-for-professionals

Grove, J. (2014) Sodexo-Times Higher Education University Lifestyle Survey results. *Times Higher Education*, 13 March. Available at: http://www.timeshighereducation.co.uk/news/sodexo-times-higher-education-university-lifestyle-survey-results/2011981.article (accessed 18 January 2015).

Health and Care Professions Council (2014) *Standards of Proficiency. Paramedics*. London: HCPC. Available at: http://www.hpc-uk.org/assets/documents/1000051CStandards_of_Proficiency_Paramedics.pdf (accessed 18 January 2015).

Lovegrove, M. (2013) *Paramedic Evidence-Based Education Project*. Buckingham: Allied Health Solutions. The Department of Health, Allied Health Professions, Professional Advisory Board.

Universities and Colleges Admissions Service website: http://www.ucas.com/

PART 2
Making the most of your academic study

3 HOW IS PARAMEDIC ACADEMIC STUDY DIFFERENT FROM OTHER SUBJECTS?

You may have friends who have studied other subjects at university and who talk about their experiences, or you might have studied at university before yourself. It is important to bear in mind that generally students who are studying health-care subjects, such as physiotherapy, midwifery, nursing and operating department practice, have a different university experience from students who study subjects where there is no clinical practice component, such as geography, English literature, social sciences and history.

Generally, students on health-care programmes have a longer academic year than other programmes, usually lasting 40–45 weeks. Health-care students also have to study whilst spending time in the clinical environment and have exposure to shift work. This chapter will relate specifically to how your study experience may be different and address some of the issues that may arise. Topics the chapter will cover include the different types of programme structure, how to manage your time and independent learning (including considering different learning styles), and, finally, how to look after your physical and mental well-being as you study, including how to cope with night shifts.

There are numerous texts available on study skills, should you require them. These should be used if you have concerns about assignment writing, referencing and accessing literature, for example. This chapter only specifically addresses the issues that a student paramedic may encounter and does not give more generic study skills advice.

Levels of study

Chapter 1 briefly introduced the importance of understanding the right level of study for you. You need to honestly appraise your academic capability and enjoyment of study. The fact is that you cannot pass a paramedic programme without passing both theoretical and practical elements. Both are equally important, so it is sensible to make sure that you are applying for the right level of study for you, whether it be a diploma, foundation degree or BSc.

Unfortunately, it is the case that for the reasons mentioned in Chapter 1 students commence paramedic study at the wrong level for them. This can potentially lead to a miserable experience. If you choose an academic level that is too challenging for you it may be that as your studies progress to a higher academic level you are constantly disappointed with your results, frustrated by your lack of progress and ultimately lose motivation and confidence. These feelings may also affect your experience and progress in the clinical environment.

It may be that you thrive in the higher education environment after not enjoying school or college. You find you become very focused on your goal and you are able to work hard and achieve very good results, the outcome all your lecturers would be aiming for. It is good to see students who initially struggled achieve their potential.

On the other hand, if you choose a lower academic level than you are capable of studying, again for the highly relevant reasons mentioned in Chapter 2, you may also end up feeling frustrated, not academically stretched and wishing you had studied at a higher level.

These varied scenarios have been included to encourage you to think a little more deeply about exactly what you want from your paramedic studies. Much of the time, especially when subjects are popular, the university process seems to be about the university choosing you, not about you choosing your university programme carefully. 'I just want a place anywhere on a paramedic programme' is not always the best approach and it may be wiser to wait, refocus, gain experience and reapply until you are totally satisfied with your choices and decision-making, as the comments in Box 3.1 explain.

As alluded to in the various comments in Box 3.1 there are numerous and wide-ranging decisions for the student to make. Paramedic studies are not *one size fits all*. The variety of programmes, in respect of structure, academic level, funding and locations, is huge and demands investigation so that you make the right choice for you. The following sections of this chapter aim to help inform your decision-making by providing some generic information on which you can build.

Box 3.1 How important is it for students to choose the right level of academic study for them?

📖 **Student paramedic response:** The first year was relatively familiar in terms of the level of study. I had just finished an access course (in order to get to uni) which was set at the same level 4 as the first year of uni. As a result I knew what amount of input I needed to give to achieve the results I was after. The jump from level 4 to 5 was a lot bigger than I expected though; in the second year the work really ramped up. It was a good learning curve though, because I learnt how much more work was needed to achieve the same results as the year before. It also gave me an idea of how much more I would need to put into my essays/dissertation in the final year when the work was at level 6.

Essays in the first year only needed one or two references per paragraph, whereas in year 3 it was closer to one per sentence! It was good though, as by year 3 I was reading around a topic so much, I was developing a much broader and deeper knowledge of it. Even though a lot of what I'd discovered didn't end up in an essay it meant that what did get put in was really relevant. You learn how to pack a lot of quality information into a small amount of words . . . which has some relevance to practice too; being able to inform hospital staff about your patient with a short, succinct, but detailed handover is a skill worth developing – year 3 essays taught me how to do that!

🎓 **Academic response:** It is important for students to choose the correct level of academic study for them. However, remember that whether studying for a diploma, foundation degree or degree, studies will all begin at the same level – level 4. Each year builds upon the last, giving you solid foundations to progress from level to level, so that by the time you reach levels 5 and 6 you will be prepared. Studying hard and getting a solid grasp of the basics in the early years of a programme will pay dividends as the level of study becomes more challenging. Remember that if you have been successful in getting on to the programme in the first place the team will have deemed you to be at a good standard. Some students will find academic work more challenging than others, but remember that academic skills can be taught if the student is prepared to listen and take the advice given to learn, improve and progress.

🚨 **Paramedic/PEd response:** One of the main elements to paramedic practice is that it is a continuous challenge; therefore, I feel that it is only right to also challenge your academic ability. However, I also acknowledge that people are different and learn in different ways and are ready for study at different times in their lives. If you find the level too challenging there are usually step-off points in programmes which will enable you to leave with academic credits. I think it is important to recognise and advocate that lower-level study should not be seen as a 'fast track' or 'easier option' to becoming a paramedic, and consideration should be put into deciding why you would need to study at a lower level, rather than why you cannot study at a higher level.

🚨 **Paramedic response:** In my experience the biggest factor for students when choosing the level of academic study they wish to undertake is that of time. It is a challenge to juggle study and work for 2 years, let alone 3. Whilst the gains in the long run are immense and really worth it, unless you are prepared to commit fully to a longer course, it may be worth considering a diploma or foundation degree and progressing to a top-up at a later date when circumstances may make this easier in some ways. You need to remember, however, that this route may have financial implications and the top-up may not be funded.

Credits

Any programme is made up of a number of academic credits. Table 3.1 explains the credit system.

Table 3.1 The academic credit system

Year	Academic level	Total credits per year	Academic award/qualification
1	4	120	Certificate
2	5	120 (240 total)	Diploma/foundation degree
3	6	120 (360 total)	BSc(Hons)

Across the course of an academic year a student will study a number of modules/units that each carry a small number of credits, usually between 10 and 60. When each of these is passed they are added together at the end of the academic year.

Generally students are required to pass 120 credits at their level of study before progressing into the next year of study. In some circumstances, students will be able to carry over some credits into the next academic year (for example, if they are waiting to resubmit a piece of work or resit an examination), but this is at the discretion of the examination board.

Generally, you will receive a letter from your institution after the formal examination board meeting has taken place, detailing your credits for the academic year and if you are required to resubmit/resit any of the modules/units the associated dates will be detailed. Again, refer to the handbook relating to your chosen programme of study for more specific detail. The programme structure will provide more specific detail about the way the programme is organised.

Clinical practice aspects of programme structure

Research the programme structure thoroughly online for the universities that you are interested in applying to. You should have the opportunity to get more detail if you are able to attend the specific university open day/evening. Paramedic and other health-care programmes have both theoretical and practice components. These can be organised in very different ways, depending on the institution. Generally, the time that you spend in clinical practice with paramedics and paramedic mentors/PEds is woven into the programme in one of three ways:

- supernumerary block placements (ambulance or mix of wider NHS placements);
- a few supernumerary clinical shifts on most weeks;
- supernumerary and employed status.

Each of these approaches will be discussed below. A word that may require some explanation is *supernumerary*; see the definition below that explains the term in relation to paramedic studies.

Definition: Supernumerary

When an ambulance crew has a student with them, there will be three of them in the vehicle. The student is additional to the clinical staff, does not form part of the crew, and is thus *supernumerary*. The student paramedic is there to observe, learn and take part in the patient's care under the direct supervision of the paramedic mentor/ PEd.

Supernumerary block placements

The term *block placement* refers to a system where students spend a period of time in university studying the theoretical and possibly some skills/simulation content; this may range between 6 and 12 weeks (the time may be ambulance-specific or a mixture of ambulance and other non-ambulance placements, depending on your programme structure). After this period in university, the student will attend the clinical area, in this case an ambulance station, to work with their paramedic mentor/ PEd and other appropriately qualified staff. At this point, the student is usually expected to mirror the shifts of their mentor/PEd, when realistically possible, and may spend up to 37 hours per seven-day week in the working environment. Some programmes may have an expectation of fewer hours per week, others may require a *full-time* commitment. If the student works fewer hours, there may be an independent study day per week.

During the course of these block placement weeks the student will also have university work to do, such as essays or examination revision, that will require submission/sitting when they attend the university for the university theory block.

Supernumerary clinical shifts on most weeks

Programmes that take this approach generally start each academic year with a week or two in university, five days per week. After this period, the student attends university one day per week and agrees two or three clinical shifts (depending on how many hours in each shift) with their mentor/ PEd for the remainder of the week. This generally leaves the student with one day for independent study and two days off each week. Each week in university the student will be focusing on specific subjects and working towards their end-of-module/unit assessment.

    ⌀ Refer to Chapter 5 for more information on subjects to be studied on paramedic programmes.

Supernumerary and employed status

Some programmes have arrangements with their partner ambulance trust where student paramedics can be employed (starting in a support worker role, not as a paramedic – note that ambulance trusts use different names for this grade of staff) after reaching a certain level of competence on the programme.

This approach generally also includes a block placement approach. Some weeks the student will be in university for up to five days per week. For some practice weeks the student will be working as a student paramedic and will have supernumerary status when on ambulance shifts. This usually means being the third person in a crew, when working in an ambulance, or the second person, if working in a car. For other weeks, the student will fulfil their role of employee for the ambulance trust, and will work, within their scope of practice, as part of a crew and not in a student paramedic role. There may be the opportunity to work in a support worker role at other times during the year, such as vacation periods. Some of these programmes have shorter holiday periods, as the student is accumulating supernumerary practice hours and also needs to work as an employee for the trust for a contracted number of hours per year.

It is important that you understand the differences and implications of each of the three structures explained above. Box 3.2 explores some thoughts about each of the approaches from the student, academic and paramedic/PEd perspective.

The comments in Box 3.2 demonstrate the flexibility of programme structures. The variety of approaches towards placement experience demonstrates the individuality that HEIs can develop in respect of their programmes. HEIs need to include the necessary subject specificity and cover the content recommended by the College of Paramedics (2014). All paramedic programmes are externally validated by the HCPC, which measures such programmes against the *Standards of Education and Training* (HCPC 2014).

Box 3.2 In your opinion what are the things a prospective student needs to consider about these approaches to paramedic study?

📖 **Academic response:** It is important to remember that the Health and Care Professions Council specifies a certain number of supernumerary hours a student must accrue in order to gain HCPC registration. Whilst it is of value for students to experience working for their trust as an employee early in the programme, they often struggle to fit in the required amount of supernumerary hours when the programme follows this route. Supernumerary block placements are of value as they allow the student to put into practice the skills and information they have acquired whilst in university. Students can concentrate on their academic studies and placement and not have to worry about fitting in 'employed' shifts.

📖 **Student paramedic response:** I worked with the system of supernumerary clinical shifts on most weeks. We were encouraged to fit two 12-hour shifts into each week alongside our uni work. By doing this we would have around 3000 placement hours by the end of our studies. The problem was that sometimes I could only book ten- or eight-hour shifts and as our studies got more intense (especially in the third year) there were times I only did one shift a week due to having so much work to do on my dissertation. Fortunately, because I had 'banked' a load of shifts in the first and second years, this worked out OK and I had more than enough hours by the end. I'd advise anyone to get loads of shifts in the first and second years so you have some breathing space during the pressure of the third year. Having said that, once the dissertation was handed in we all booked as many shifts as we could to boost our confidence, as we were all acutely aware that we would be 'on the road' within a few weeks.

🚨 **Paramedic mentor/PEd response:** Whilst placement/supernumerary hours are focused around working actual shifts with a mentor, this does not mean there won't be ample opportunity for students to work on coursework, exam revision, etc. I have always explained to students that this is not an either-or situation. Being on placement quite often gives an excellent opportunity for mentors to help students with their university work and it is particularly useful to link theory with practice. Whilst it is not feasible for a student to write an assignment whilst on shift, it is possible to advance the theoretical aspects of the job by exposure to and discussion around the different conditions encountered.

☞ **Academic response:** Supernumerary placements are of great benefit to students, allowing them maximum contact with their mentors and opportunity to practise their skills under direct supervision, which is not always the case where students make up part of an operational crew, e.g. some foundation degree programmes. As part of an operational crew, students will often end up driving the patient to hospital, when challenging cases are being treated in the back of the vehicle, thus missing valuable opportunities to manage these cases under direct supervision.

🕴 **Paramedic mentor/PEd response:** There are positives and negatives to both types of clinical practice facilitation; however, the main points to consider are continuity, exposure and time management. In paramedic practice each patient varies considerably from the last, making it impossible to plan for what you will see and how frequently you will see things. By having continual exposure (two or three clinical shifts per week) you are more 'available', and this reduces the feeling of being pressured into seeing as much as possible in the short space of time, a potential negative of block placement. I think it depends on what you are used to; whatever the system used by your university, you will get used to it. Additionally, with continual placements you are developing your time management ability, as you need to plan academic study into your working week, whilst maintaining a healthy work–life balance.

☞ **Academic response:** I have taught on programmes where students are required to undertake supernumerary block placements, parts of employment and programmes where students do supernumerary shifts each week alongside university work. Each approach has positives and negatives. Some students struggle to separate their employed ambulance service role from their role of being a student, others struggle with completing university work while on a block clinical placement, and others struggle with managing shift patterns and university days. For all of these struggles, many students just enjoy being in the clinical area, whatever form that takes. Prospective students need to be aware that these variations exist and think about which approach will best suit their learning approach and personal needs.

Note: All programmes are different, in respect of the amount of practice hours that students are expected to accumulate across the duration of their programme, whether that is 2 or 3 years. The *minimum* number of practice hours that require evidencing for eligibility to register with the HCPC is 750 hours per year, across the duration of your programme. With a three-year programme the student needs to evidence a minimum of 2250 (3 × 750) hours in total. The College of Paramedics (2014: 35) 'stipulates that 50 percent of the programme should be undertaken in the clinical practice setting', and 'a maximum of 5 percent of the recommended practice placement hours can be used to assess paramedic competencies in the simulated environment' (2014: 37).

The following parts of this chapter refer to study skills and aspects of self-care that are particularly pertinent to the student paramedic. These parts of the chapter should be used in conjunction with a general study skills text.

Managing and planning your studies

As you can imagine, the programme structure is likely to have a big impact on the way you manage and plan your studies. Your experience of working independently may also have an impact on your success, or lack thereof, at planning and managing your studies. To understand the amount of self-directed study that is required for any programme, look at the amount of learning hours allocated for each module. You will not be taught everything you need to know in class, and you will see that face-to-face taught sessions make up only a small percentage of the allocated learning hours. It is important that you develop as an independent learner as well as an independent practitioner. Do not underestimate how much work is involved! The student comment below demonstrates how organised, disciplined and structured it is possible to be.

Student paramedic comment: I thought of my study days in terms of three blocks of time – morning, afternoon, evening. I would then study during two of those blocks and take the third one off. I found I studied best either in the morning or evening, so I would take afternoons out and do something to recharge the batteries. You might study better during morning and afternoon, or afternoon and evening – whatever suits you, if you take two blocks for study and one for yourself you'll get the work done and keep yourself refreshed.

This section explores some of the realities of each of the placement systems explained above.

Supernumerary block placement

Prior to your block placement, the university staff will deliver much of the material required for you to complete whatever module/unit you are studying and the associated assessment. Now, however, you will need to undertake additional reading and research the resources that are introduced at university. As a student you may have competing demands when you are at university full-time for a period of weeks, such as peer pressure to socialise and/or having to work in the evenings/weekends. Before going to clinical placement it would be wise to borrow library texts (if they are not available as e-books or online articles) and have a clear idea of what is required in terms of the assessment for this part of the programme. While you are on clinical placement it may be difficult to co-ordinate shifts with the commitments of your lecturers, if additional appointments are required. With this type of programme structure you need to be extremely disciplined with independent study and keep working towards both academic and clinical assessment that will be assessed by your paramedic mentor/PEd.

Supernumerary clinical shifts on most weeks

This approach usually incorporates an independent study day on most weeks, in addition to university attendance and generally two (12-hour) or three (8-hour) supernumerary clinical shifts per week. The student will generally have weekly contact with the university lecturers and paramedic mentors/PEds. This should enable the student to discuss and clarify any issues that occur while on placement with university staff quite easily and also to continuously focus what has happened on the road with the theory discussed in lectures. Theoretically this should make planning and managing your studies easier. However, in reality some students are not disciplined enough to utilise the independent study time successfully. Some students struggle with the concept of working independently, deciding what it is they need to study. This may be your first experience of not being told exactly what to study and focus upon. University lecturers should be able to provide guidance on this, but only if you report you are having difficulty planning and managing your studies.

Supernumerary and employed status

As with supernumerary block placement, this approach will potentially entail several weeks away from the university campus, so diligence and a disciplined approach to study is essential. Accessing resources from university is generally not an issue, with remote access and many texts now available as e-books. It can become quite complex for the student in respect of assessment in practice when mixing supernumerary and employment status. The nature of the paramedic role is one of unplanned and often unexpected experiences, so practice assessment can rarely be planned. It can be quite frustrating for many students if during the course of their employed time they experience an episode of patient care that requires assessment in their student role. If the student is part of a crew, being paid and not in a supernumerary role, no assessment is generally allowed, as the student will not be working with their mentor/PEd or being supervised. Generally this assessment should only take place when they are working with their mentor/PEd; this is generally not the case when they are working shifts during employed weeks.

No matter what the type of placement arrangement, it is important that you ensure that placement assessment documentation is completed in a timely manner, as it may not always be possible to obtain signatures or feedback after the event.

You would be wise to research and read a study skills book that makes sense to you and that you find informative. Studying at an HEI will be different from school or college; it is much more about personal responsibility and commitment to your studies. In addition to taught lectures, other forms of teaching and learning will be used, such as group work, presentations and simulation.

Learning outcomes

Each module or unit will have a set of learning outcomes. Each student must meet these specific learning outcomes. The assessment task, whether it be coursework, an assignment or an examination, will be designed to test the student's competence in meeting the learning outcomes. The lectures, seminars, workshops, skills sessions and guided study will be focused on delivering and discussing material that is specific to the learning outcomes. Students will also be provided with information about the assessment task and deadlines for submission of work (or examination date) and the subsequent planning and management of work is the students' responsibility. Any materials given to the cohort while at university are generally introductory, and the students will be expected to undertake additional reading and expand their knowledge sufficiently in order to excel at the assessment task.

Time management

Students on health-care courses often have lots of balls in the air that they need to juggle. Many students will have family commitments, the pressure of working part-time hours in addition to meeting the demands of shift work as a student paramedic. It is easy for studying and independent study to take a back seat in favour of prioritising what needs to be done now. The inevitable consequence is that a submission date looms and you are trying to study at times when you are not productive, not reading sufficiently and rushing your work in order to meet the deadline. By knowing your learning style and study habits (both good and bad) you may be able to make a positive impact. Managing your time more efficiently may help.

Reflection: points to consider

At what time of day do you most enjoy studying?

At what time of day are you at your most productive?

Do you plan your studies to coincide with the answers you have given to the questions above?

With so many aspects to consider, the student paramedic may benefit from planning their studies on a weekly basis. No two students are the same, so each should plan their studies to suit their needs and make the most of times in the day when they work efficiently and are at their most productive. It is also important to plan in leisure time, socialising and relaxing activities. Many students find this approach works for them and their planner becomes their support network, telling them what to do and when to do it. It generally enables you to be more disciplined, not leave your work until the last minute and, gradually each week, work towards your final goal of a completed piece of work that is of the standard you wish to submit, or fully prepare for an examination. In Box 3.3 students, academics and mentors/PEds give a variety of opinions on time management.

Box 3.3 What advice would you give to student paramedics about time management?

Year 1 students:

📖 Try to start assignments early, to get the most out of lectures.

📖 Make sure you plan your study time. Don't be tempted to schedule placement/other work when you should be reading/studying.

Year 2/3 students:

📖 At times when you don't have assignments, don't stop reading. Do preparation for the next term in your holidays, not tons, just a little, so you know what is coming when you return to uni.

📖 Get into the habit of additional reading early. Things like anatomy and physiology are essential to placement and understanding what is happening to your patients, so you can always read that and learn something you didn't know. And you will be asked questions on it by your mentor/PEd.

🎓 **Academic response:** Start your assignment early and make sure you send an assignment plan to your tutor. This will ensure you are thinking along the right lines and haven't wasted valuable time writing about the wrong things or tackling things in the wrong way.

When it comes to studying for tests and exams, ask your tutor in which areas you should direct your revision. Again, this will save valuable time which may have been spent revising the wrong things.

If you feel you may be falling behind, do not leave things to get out of hand. Speak to your tutors and to your student support officer who will be able to help.

Paramedic mentor/PEd response: Just because you are out on placement does not mean you cannot continue your academic studies. Not all shifts are busy, and a lot of time can be spent on standby. I have always used this time to work with my students on their academic studies. This has always proven invaluable to the student and in a way gives bonus study time that has not necessarily been timetabled in. Over the years in this bonus time I have been able to take a look at assignments, clarify areas students did not fully understand, research specific conditions we may have encountered, and work through question and answer sessions.

Academic response: Don't forget that your module handbook/ guide should clearly explain what the assessment criteria are. Read all module material carefully to ensure that you are fully aware of what is required. Also be especially aware that there may be considerable amounts of reflection etc. hidden in practice portfolios.

Paramedic mentor/PEd response: Time management is vital, pre-planning to ensure you have sufficient time to complete academic assignments is a priority, and continuing your own development with critical reading, reflection and independent study is a must. In respect of practice, time management is also important to ensure you arrive at work clean, punctual and with the resources required to carry out your shifts. You also need to make sure that you have eaten, that you sleep well and that you maintain a healthy body and mind by ensuring you manage time to ensure days of rest and relaxation too. Getting into a habit of effective time management at the beginning of study can only be of benefit and helps to ease the pressure of the demands of your programme.

Planning your study is one aspect of learning; it is also important to understand that your learning style may affect your approach to learning.

Learning styles: what type of learner are you?

As individuals we learn in different ways, that is, we have different learning styles. Your learning style is an important aspect of understanding more about yourself, and it is important to appreciate that the way subjects are taught may not always appeal to your preferred learning style. As a student, it is easy to *switch off* when you encounter a teaching style that you find uncomfortable or not to your taste. As an adult learner it is important to recognise the reasons why this may be the case and work on a strategy to enable you to get the most from all teaching strategies.

This is not a new concept, and the work of Kolb (1974) and subsequently Honey and Mumford (1986) is seminal in the discussion of learning styles. There are many derivatives of their original work and some free online tools to assist you in self-assessment of your learning style. An understanding of what Kolb (1974) and Honey and Mumford (1986) proposed is important for the student to begin any self-assessment.

Kolb (1974) suggested that we all learn through a sequence of activities which are related. He suggested there are four stages to the activities:

1   An experience
2   Observations and reflections about the experience
3   A theoretical proposition about the event
4   Active experimentation and testing – by further action and testing the accuracy of the theoretical view of what has happened. The person will then circle the spiral of learning again from stage 1.

Kolb's (1974) learning theory has specific pertinence to student paramedics and their related practice experiences. Many paramedic programmes also encompass the use of reflection in trying to make sense of students' practice experiences.

The evidence-based clinician will also understand the theoretical information related to the practice experience and have reflected on their handling or performance of the event. They will also have an action plan should they encounter a similar event in the future. This is not exactly stage 4 of Kolb's (1974) model, as encounters with patients cannot be 'staged' and are generally not exactly the same. Nonetheless, the model is relevant to the world of the student paramedic.

Kolb's (1974) model has been critiqued by Honey and Mumford (1986) as being simplistic and not taking into account the learning styles of the student. They proposed that individuals will spend different amounts of time at each of the four stages of Kolb's model, depending on the way in which they learn. For example, some individuals will reflect more than others (stage 2), some will spend an inordinate amount of time reading and investigating the theory around the experience (stage 3) but not think much about their own actions, and others will carry on to the next experience without spending much time at all on stages 2 and 3.

Honey and Mumford (1986) proposed that there are four types of learners:

1 Activist
2 Reflector
3 Theorist
4 Pragmatist.

Tables 3.2–3.5 outline the characteristics and teaching styles/activities that each type of learner will learn most from, as proposed by Honey and Mumford (1986).

Table 3.2 Activist characteristics and teaching activities

Characteristics	Teaching activities
People who learn by doing	Problem-solving
Need to get their hands dirty	Group discussion
Dive in with both feet first	Puzzles
Open-minded approach to learning	Competitions
Involve themselves fully and without bias in new experiences	Role play
	Explore lots of ideas all at once to come up with one or two that help solve a problem

Source: adapted from Honey and Mumford (1986).

Table 3.3 Reflector characteristics and teaching activities

Characteristics	Teaching activities
Learn by observing and thinking about what has happened	Paired discussion
May avoid leaping in and prefers to watch from the sidelines	Self-analysis questionnaires
Prefer to stand back and view new experiences from a number of perspectives	Personality questionnaires
Collect data and take time to work towards an appropriate conclusion	Time out
	Observing activities
	Feedback from others
	Interviews
	Coaching

Source: adapted from Honey and Mumford (1986).

Table 3.4 Theorist characteristics and teaching activities

Characteristics	Teaching activities
Like to understand the theory behind the actions	Models
Need models, concepts and facts in order to engage in learning	Statistics
Prefer to analyse and synthesise	Stories
Develop new information into a systematic and logical theory	Quotes
	Background information
	Applying theories

Source: adapted from Honey and Mumford (1986).

Table 3.5 Pragmatist characteristics and teaching activities

Characteristics	Teaching activities
Need to be able to see how to put learning into practice in the real world	Time to think about how to apply learning to reality
Abstract concepts are of limited use	Case studies
Need to see a way of putting ideas into action in their lives	Problem-solving
Experimenters, trying out new ideas, theories and techniques to see if they work	Discussion

Source: adapted from Honey and Mumford (1986).

The activist is generally enthusiastic about anything new and will try anything once. Activists have a tendency to act first and consider the consequences later. In terms of completing projects, they enjoy the ideas stage and new challenges, but once an action plan is in place to complete the project the activist will become bored and lose interest in the implementation and completion of the task. If you recognise these characteristics in yourself and are well prepared, you may be able to find additional ways to maintain your interest. A student paramedic who is naturally an activist needs to be aware of the tendency to rush in, especially when patients are involved, as this may not always be the right or most appropriate action. If you know this is your natural tendency you should force yourself to think before diving in. The activist is someone who needs to be busy all the time (this can be quite tiring for others) and may need to be controlled in a practice situation to prevent mistakes being made.

Student paramedics who are natural reflectors may find practice experience or learning in simulation initially quite challenging and in some situations quite stressful. If your natural tendency is to observe and analyse information, you may need to make a conscious effort to push yourself to get involved. It is also important to be aware of how you may appear to others (family members, colleagues, mentors). Natural reflectors would not want to be thought of as unenthusiastic and disinterested.

A natural theorist will enjoy the academic aspects of study and probably find independent study quite enjoyable. Theorists need to be mindful, when in practice, about the most appropriate time and place to be asking questions. If you are a natural theorist you may find the practice environment quite constraining – you may have to wait to go and investigate a subject area, such as a certain medical condition, as you will not necessarily have the resources available to do all the reading and investigation that you wish to do at the time. A student paramedic with this natural tendency may have to work on the person-to-person skills of the paramedic role, such as communication and skills development.

A student with a pragmatist natural tendency may find it difficult to relate the theory being taught in the classroom to the clinical area. If you have strong pragmatist traits you may find practice more interesting, as you will witness your mentors/PEds take action, but you may need your mentor to explain the theory behind the care being given to a patient in order for you to understand the link between theory and practice.

Remember that the learning styles described in Tables 3.2–3.5 are generally not exclusive; you may identify with several characteristics from all four tables. Most of us fall naturally into one of the four categories, but we will also possess characteristics from the other learning styles. Having an understanding of predominant learning styles may enable you to work on and develop what you may perceive as other useful attributes. This should also help you to develop a sense of who you are which should be useful to your overall development as a student paramedic, in both an academic and practice environment, as reinforced by comments in Box 3.4.

Another learning preference that is worthwhile exploring is the visual auditory reading (and writing) kinaesthetic (VARK) model of learning styles, which Fleming (2001) developed. He developed his four styles from the area of neurolinguistic programming, where the previous VAK model was used. Fleming (2001) added a further approach, that of reading and writing (R). This approach has been designed around the concept that learners use four ways to receive and learn new information, one or two of the approaches being dominant for each individual:

- V = Visual
- A = Auditory
- R = Reading and writing
- K = Kinaesthetic (movement).

For the purposes of this text only three approaches (VAK) will be discussed, as reading and writing approaches are more appropriately discussed in respect of school-age children, not adult learners. Understanding which approach you prefer will enable you to use the suggestions included in Tables 3.6–3.8 when studying in the academic arena or working independently.

Box 3.4 What are the benefits of knowing your learning style?

🎓 **Academic response:** The different subjects you will study will naturally lend themselves to certain learning styles. For example, anatomy and physiology is an academic subject usually taught in lecture format, particularly if the cohort is large. Whilst the lecturer may like to take a different approach to this subject, it is sometimes simply impossible due to logistics, e.g. room size, time available.

This form of teaching would appeal to the natural theorist, while the pragmatist may not enjoy it. Knowing your own personal learning style will help you to understand that it may not be the subject matter you do not engage with but the style of delivery. If this is the case you will be able to work out ways in which to undertake self-study of the subject that will make it more enjoyable. For example, a lecture on the pathophysiology of myocardial infarction could be built upon by discussing this with your mentor after attending such an incident and seeing it in reality. In this way you can see how this has relevance to practice and relate it to the underpinning theory. This approach would appeal to those with a different learning style.

Most programmes have a range of study and activities that will appeal, at some stage, to all learning styles.

📖 **Student paramedic response:** Early in the programme we did an exercise to discover what learning styles we most related to. This was useful in that it helped make us more aware of how we could tailor our personal study in such a way as to get the most out of it. As a visual/kinaesthetic learner, I found watching my mentor carrying out clinical procedures then copying what he did was far easier than reading about how to do them and then trying myself. As a result I made sure I was in a position to see how things were done by the different paramedics I worked with on shifts. I would then check with my mentor that I was doing these skills correctly and get his input too. I still read up on skills etc., it just meant I learnt them in a way that worked for me.

Table 3.6 highlights the main points for consideration by students who prefer learning visually. Visual learning can be divided into two subsections, linguistic and spatial. If you prefer the visual approach to learning you may benefit from taking notes during lectures, using drawings to supplement your notes and then rereading them afterwards for clarification. Think about the value of converting your lecture notes into a more visual reminder, such as concept maps, charts and illustrations.

Table 3.6 Characteristics of visual learners

Visual – linguistic	Visual – spatial
Learn through written language, e.g. reading and writing	Have difficulty with the written language
Remember what has been written down	Do better with charts, demonstrations, videos and other visual materials
Like to write down directions	Easily visualise faces and places by using their imagination
Pay better attention to lectures if they watch them	Seldom get lost in new surroundings

Auditory learners have characteristics like those listed in Table 3.7. If you tend to learn more when an auditory style of learning is used you will benefit from lecturers or mentors summarising what has happened. You can help yourself by writing questions about the subject content from your notes and will find this an easier way to learn. Mentors/PEds and lecturers find that auditory learners enjoy being questioned and need longer to debrief.

Table 3.7 Characteristics of auditory learners

Often talk to themselves
May move their lips and read out loud
May have difficulty with reading and writing tasks
Often do better talking to a colleague
May benefit from using a tape recorder, in order to hear what was said in lectures

Kinaesthetic learners often learn more if they are able to move and touch objects while learning. The characteristics are therefore divided into kinaesthetic (movement) and tactile (touch) in Table 3.8. If you are this type of learner you will relish the practical elements of paramedic study as it enables you to keep on the move and use your hands. A kinaesthetic learner will enjoy and learn best when lectures are more practical in nature and involve moving around the classroom. Many student paramedics will categorise themselves as kinaesthetic learners, but students must also be aware of and use strategies to help them apply themselves in different learning situations.

Table 3.8 Characteristics of kinaesthetic learners

Kinaesthetic (movement)	Tactile (touch)
Will lose concentration without movement around them	May take notes for no other reason than being able to touch external surfaces, e.g. the pen, paper
Take notes by drawing pictures, doodling, diagrams	Use colour highlighters
When reading, will scan the material first and then focus in on the details, so need a while to read	When reading, will scan the material first and then focus in on the details, so need a while to read

A large variety of approaches to learning are used on paramedic programmes, but not all strategies will suit all students. It is important that you do what you can to learn about yourself and develop learning and study strategies to make the most of all the information presented to you.

If you have a good understanding of your learning style you will be in a better position to look out for yourself.

Looking after yourself

The career you have chosen is one of unpredictability, varied stress, shift work, and is often physically and mentally demanding. In order to achieve any longevity in a career as a paramedic (which could be 30–40 years in length), it is of the utmost importance to look after yourself. This section considers physical and mental well-being separately, but they are inextricably linked.

Student paramedic comment: Our programme was hard work. Really hard work! Dealing with night shifts and unpleasant or disturbing call-outs, whilst swotting for exams and trying to work out where Harvard referencing wanted you to put a comma or a full stop in your essay references, took its toll on all of us. It's important to look after yourself. You need rest time as much as study time. In fact you won't learn as well if you don't rest well. It's all about having the right balance. Whatever equals rest and relaxation for you, make sure you schedule it into your week. I'd suggest getting out of the house and away from the computer and doing something which has nothing to do with 'work'.

I found early morning runs were great for keeping physically and mentally healthy. If I was under pressure from an essay deadline or after a difficult shift, going for a run cleared my head and refreshed me.

Physical well-being

Will I get ill?

As the comments in Box 3.5 clearly articulate, as a student paramedic you will be exposed to people who are ill and you will also be expected to undertake shift work, which may be a new experience. Both of these will be challenging to your immune system. Minor illnesses are usually more prevalent in the first year of a programme, as your immune system takes time to protect itself from the range and variety of bacteria, viruses and diseases you are exposed to.

To sleep or not too sleep?

Shift work is a unique experience, and though most shifts are manageable, the struggles some people face with night shifts can be difficult to explain to anyone who has never experienced them. Many health-care workers struggle with sleeping when on night work, as the comments in Box 3.6 illustrate, and this is something that student paramedics often worry about when they first commence a programme of study.

Box 3.5 What would be your advice for minimising the potential for illness?

📖 **Senior student response:** Obviously don't make illness more likely. Use infection control procedures – gloves, hand washing, etc. – but try not to walk in with an anti-radioactive suit on! There is self-protection, then there's overreaction. Keeping your immune system strong and healthy will lower your chances of catching bugs.

🎓 **Academic response:** I would recommend eating foods rich in vitamin C or adding a supplement, prior to placement exposure. You will be ill, certainly in year 1, don't worry, once you are a registered paramedic you will have an immune system to be proud of!

🔦 **Paramedic mentor/PEd response:** Expect to catch every bug going in your first year of placement. This is normal until your immune system develops, and shift work doesn't help. Disruption of sleep patterns can lower the immune system, as can stress. This will get better as your immune system adapts and you get used to shift work. Eat well and sleep well when you can. Make sure you leave time for yourself. Nothing lowers the immune system and affects health as much as stress.

🔦 **Paramedic mentor/PEd response:** Firstly and most importantly, personal hygiene needs to take priority, short nails, showering, clean uniform, hair tied up; however, this needs to be done in conjunction with effective clinical hygiene, the appropriate use of personal protective equipment and strict hand hygiene. Likewise, it is important to ensure vaccinations are kept up to date and you adhere to standard precautions, such as the safe handling of the disposal of sharps, segregating linen and cleaning equipment. Eating a healthy balanced diet, drinking plenty of fluids and ensuring a regular and healthy sleep pattern is important. Inadvertently, exposure to illness and catching the occasional one will assist in developing an immune system that rejects illnesses that you come across most often!

Box 3.6 What is your advice for coping with shift work and sleeping?

📖 **Student paramedic response:** Everyone is different. I personally find sleeping for three hours in the afternoon helpful before a night shift. Then, after a shift, sleep from 09.00 or 10.00 until two hours before your shift starts. You need to learn about your body.

🎓 **Academic response:** Contrary to popular belief, all your lecturers will have experienced shift work at some point in their careers – so we do understand and we may have some helpful suggestions if you are finding it hard, but you need to talk to us. Some people hate it, some tolerate it, some love it – you need to make up your own mind. One thing is for sure, you cannot do this job without having to do shifts and night work. I only ever slept for five hours after any night shift, usually from 08.00 to 13.00, and that is a long time to be awake – until 08.00 the following morning. During waking hours I felt like a bit of a zombie; although I was capable of functioning, sometimes it felt like I wasn't really there, a feeling difficult to explain. Sleep when your body tells you it wants to (but generally not during your night shift!) even if it is only for an hour. Sleeping in the heat of the summer is worse, due to the light, noise and having to sleep with a window open – generally student paramedics do not experience this as they are on leave for most of the hot summer weather.

🚨 **Paramedic mentor/PEd response:** Shift work initially is a shock to the system. My best advice would be get to know your own body clock well! You will soon learn what your body needs to function. Some helpful hints would be having a lie-in the morning before a night shift or getting some sleep in the afternoon leading up to a night shift, then ensuring you eat accordingly either overnight or when you return home and getting sleep the following day. Get some sleep after your final night but allow yourself time to tire throughout the day so you can still sleep that night, so your body returns to a normal pattern. Blacking out curtains, showering before bed, not drinking caffeine near the end of your shift could all help with the process.

🚨 **Paramedic mentor/PEd response:** Adapting to night shifts is always a challenge for those who haven't experienced this before. Changes of shift patterns due to the rota you are working is particularly difficult. Changing from days to nights or vice versa was one of the things I found most difficult. I would just get used to working nights and find it was time to change over onto days. Most people get used to shift work over time. If your body tells you it is time to sleep take notice of it, even if this may be at an unconventional time. 'Power snoozing' is of immense value, and even 20 minutes can revitalise you. After 18 years in the job I always joke that I can fall asleep to order – immediately and anywhere!

As you will note from the range of comments above, every individual develops their own coping strategy. The most important thing is to be open-minded and try several strategies until you find a way that suits you.

Food – what to eat

Some student paramedics may not be used to preparing and cooking their own meals. Learn the basics of eating healthily before you start your programme, if you have to prepare your own meals and have not done so before. Eating healthily is important in maintaining physical fitness, so that everyday aspects of the paramedic role can be carried out safely, without danger to yourself or the patient, such as moving and handling. It also plays a part in maintaining mental health. Box 3.7 provides some ideas.

Box 3.7 Is eating healthily important for student paramedics? What advice would you give?

📖 **Student response:** There is no excuse during times you are at uni. On placement it is sometimes difficult. Often you only get one meal break and not a lot of time to think healthily; we often snack. I have no problem with snacking. The problem I have is with what we choose to snack. I find myself, having not eaten for a long period of time, just eating something sweet – to get my blood sugar up – and things like crisps. Not the best for long-term health. The food we can nibble on throughout the day and stay fit varies hugely. I would suggest nuts, fruit, malt loaf, sesame snacks, fruit bars, for example. I worked in fitness before this career choice and know that nothing makes me feel as good as being healthy and not hungry.

🎓 **Academic response:** Eating healthily should not be a problem when in university but can become a challenge when on placement, particularly on night shifts when your body cannot work out whether it is breakfast or dinner time. Taking your own healthy packed lunch to work can be of benefit and will mean you do not miss a meal if you cannot return to base.

🚨 **Paramedic mentor/PEd response:** The pressures of being a student and living alone for possibly the first time, being responsible for your own shopping, cooking and being restricted with time can all lead to eating a very different diet. Getting into a routine to plan meals and eat healthily isn't that difficult once you start, and although many people will say it is hard to plan meals when working shift work, I disagree! You can still find time to prepare healthy foods, and there are plenty of healthy snacks that don't need to be put in a fridge that will see you through the day! As for sugar rushes, there are still healthy options available, and chocolate isn't that bad once in a while! If you start a routine it soon becomes the norm, so start healthy eating at the beginning and you won't look back!

🚨 **Paramedic mentor/PEd response:** Beware the 4a.m. chocolate attack! Without fail I would always crave something sweet at this time on night shifts. I would always take a pack up to work, so even if I did not manage to get back to base I could eat. This is far better than relying on getting back to base to microwave what you have brought or grabbing fast food. By taking my own pack up I have always been able to find time to eat on shift when I have been hungry. The only downside with this way of working is that the speed at which you eat will change. It is a standing joke in my family that my plate is always cleared first – years of working with the 'grab it while you have time' outlook!

Mental well-being

You will face some extremely taxing (both physically and mentally) encounters with patients and families during the course of your studies and long afterwards. It is commonly accepted that it is impossible to prepare for every eventuality, but there are some things that may help you to develop an awareness of your own mental health and well-being and manage the various situations in positive ways. As individuals we have many aspects to our personalities, and what will affect one person may not affect their friend in the same way. Appreciating each other's differences and being able to recognise stress, firstly in yourself and then in others, is one major starting point. Conversely, it may be that what other people think is a major issue does not bother you. As the student comment below highlights, the patient encounters that you think will bother you are often the conditions you see more often.

Student paramedic comment: Sometimes you may go to a job which affects you more than others. For me it wasn't the trauma jobs (not that we go to that many!), it was some of the jobs where people were struggling with huge social or mental health issues which got to me most. At other times the academic workload may start to feel unmanageable, or it could be a life event that happens to a relative or friend outside of uni that has an effect on you.

Lots of things can conspire together to put you under a lot of pressure. If this starts to affect your day-to-day life it is best to go and talk to someone. As students our first line of defence was talking with each other – a problem shared and all that. For bigger things, talking with our programme leader and lecturers was always beneficial. Our university also gave us access to free professional counselling services if we had issues which we needed help with. These could be accessed anonymously via student services, with appointments fitting in with students' schedules. I know that some students used this service and found it very helpful. The important thing is that if you find things getting on top of you, you needn't suffer in silence, go and talk to someone you trust. The help is there if you need it.

⌀ Refer to Chapter 12 for more on difficult calls and Chapter 13 for more on resilience.

Reflection

The importance of reflecting on issues should not be underestimated. Reflection happens naturally as part of the day. Within programmes it may be addressed specifically as a subject, part of an assignment, portfolio or other academic work. This section focuses on reflection as a means of maintaining positive mental health. Some people find it difficult to reflect; the process can be quite challenging, but generally becomes easier the more you begin to understand yourself and the role that you are entering as a paramedic. This chapter does not attempt to explore reflection in any depth, but there are some suggested texts listed at the end of this chapter. In fact there are numerous texts to choose from. Take some time to explore the subject and start to understand more about reflection.

Part of the learning process is reviewing things that have happened to you, whether it be in the classroom, in practice, with your mentor/PEd or when caring for a patient. Making sense of whatever is bothering you (or deciding that it does not and never will make sense) is the key to mental well-being, as Case Study 3.1 demonstrates. As health-care professionals we constantly discuss the importance of communication. This applies to us, not just patients and families. We need to recognise the value of talking to each other, our loved ones, professional counsellors if that is what we require, without experiencing reproach or stigma.

CASE STUDY 3.1

Andy was four months into year 1 of his paramedic studies. While on shift with his mentor they attended a road traffic accident, involving the death (on scene) of a middle-aged man. Andy talked to his mentor about what had happened and the fact this was the first traumatic incident he had been to and first dead person he had seen. Andy thought about all that had happened and was personally reflecting on his experiences. He experienced no adverse reactions, such as insomnia, nightmares or loss of appetite. He was managing well at this point. Three days later he received a call from his home town, some miles away from university, to tell him that one of his best friends was dead, having been involved in a road traffic accident (he died at the scene). As more details emerged, it soon became apparent that Andy's friend's accident was within an hour of the one he had attended, albeit hundreds of miles away. Andy tried to learn more of the detail and began comparing the two incidents. He recalled minute details of his patient; this served to make his patient real and Andy obsessed about the same thing happening to his friend. On lengthy discussion, debriefing and reflection, Andy realised that he required time away from his studies to make sense of what had happened, be with his family and friends and reflect. Andy used writing as one means of helping him cope. His account was personal to him, but enabled him to think about and explore more detail than he says he achieved by talking. Andy slowly came to terms with the ordeal, but never did understand why this had happened. Andy returned to be successful at his studies.

Case Study 3.1 demonstrates the vulnerability in each of us, and our ability to cope with extreme situations will be different for each of us. What is important is that we recognise that what we are feeling is unusual and becoming an issue, talk to someone and take action to improve our well-being. Andy's experience is clearly disturbing, but reflection and other coping mechanisms helped him manage his bereavement. Box 3.8 describes the use of reflection more generally and recalls some occasions where reflection has helped practitioners.

> **Box 3.8 Can you give an example of a situation where reflection was a useful tool for you to use? Did you appreciate the value of reflection when you were a student?**
>
> 📖 **Student response:** I went to a job in the first year which involved a homeless street drinker from eastern Europe who was fitting. The patient was very difficult and abusive. The crew I was with were sure he was not truly having a seizure but was simply trying to get out of the cold. However, they explained that just because they were suspicious of this, and had seen people do this many times, they could be wrong in their opinion and had an overriding duty of care to take him into the Emergency Department (ED) for further assessment and treatment. At ED the man continued to be difficult. Afterwards we all felt quite annoyed that the man had appeared to be manipulating the situation by using the ED as a place to keep warm and sleep.
>
> I went home and did a reflective study into this job and ended up changing my attitude towards the homeless man as I found out more about the situation he was in and the likely events which led to it. I also examined my own attitude and feelings about the job and why I had felt that way. By the end of the reflective process I felt I had a greater perspective on the job and came to the honest conclusion that had I been in the same situation as the homeless man I probably

would have done the same thing as he did – there but for the grace of God and all that.

Consequently, whilst I may have developed a healthy scepticism in relation to some jobs we go to, I would now say that that scepticism is accompanied by a greater degree of understanding, empathy and appreciation of why people sometimes see the ambulance service as a short-term answer to some of their social problems.

Academic response: My first introduction to structured reflection was as a student myself, and I was initially not enamoured. Topics for reflection were specified in advance, and I was forced to reflect on some situations that were better left alone. This should never be the case and students should not have to 'dig up' disturbing instances that they have dealt with in their own way and moved on from. It is up to you what you choose to reflect on, and in many cases you will find yourself doing this naturally. It is second nature for us to talk through the jobs that didn't run so smoothly and discuss what we could have done to improve things. Structured reflection is the next step up from this and is an invaluable tool to improve practice, discover ourselves and find out more about certain presenting complaints. The frameworks used should not be viewed as rigid but should rather be used as a prompt for pointing out in what areas and in what way it may be useful to direct our reflection.

Academic response: It is true that sometimes students do not know what to reflect on, when asked to do so in a classroom situation or for an assignment. Be guided by knowing yourself. Is there something that is keeping you awake at night, a nagging feeling that you could have done more on a job, wondering what happened to that patient? I would say all of these are indicators that things are bothering you. Why not try using a reflective model to help prompt you to think about each event in an ordered and less chaotic way than your brain may do at inappropriate times of the day, such as 4a.m.! Just try it, it may well help you.

Paramedic mentor/PEd response: I used a reflective model too but I also used PowerPoint to reflect, still following a model of reflection but using slides to demonstrate my thoughts, feelings and abilities which I could then talk through and present to my peers. This way, I felt I got more out of it. After attending a cardiac arrest of a young person, writing it all down was fine and it demonstrated what I had done, but having the ability to reflect through discussion via a presentation allowed for others to share their views and opinions with me. This helped me to understand and explore my thoughts and feelings in more detail, as I had an understanding of how others would have processed this incident as well. Reflection was extremely beneficial to me throughout my study and I still use it frequently. I strongly believe reflection is the key to developing myself and improving my abilities. I also advocate the importance of reflection to students, and how it is useful for self-development, but also important in being able to maintain a healthy state of mind, as you can use it to reflect on your feelings.

Paramedic mentor/PEd response: It is vitally important to recognise that reflection does not necessarily have to take a formal, structured form. Some of the most valuable reflections throughout the course of my career have been informal and have taken place with my colleagues/crew in the crew room. This 'work family' are in the unique position of understanding exactly where you are coming from. This informal form of reflection has as much validity as structured 'academic' reflection, and its power should not be underestimated. The important thing is that you are beginning to develop a reflective personality, something that will stand you in good stead in the future.

It may be that you encounter something during or after your studies that you are not able to understand or manage successfully on your own or with family support. Sometimes individuals need specialist help, in exactly the same way we may need specialist physical care. In such situations students need to access appropriate services.

Accessing services

Most programmes have a handbook where there is considerable information – read it! It will probably include a section on the roles of people within the programme team at your university. This brief section highlights some useful roles within university teams that may be able to help.

Personal tutor/lecturer

Usually programme teams will allocate students to individual lecturers in the team to act as personal tutors for the duration of the student's studies. This role is usually classified as pastoral, meaning this should be the person you go to if you want to discuss anything that may not be specifically related to programme content or subject specific information. Your personal tutor will be able to signpost specific, specialised assistance, should it be required. A personal tutor is a role created to help students navigate their way through university systems, procedures and policies and to provide help and assistance. This role is invaluable, if students feel able to talk to their personal tutor. Most universities will provide a role description – find this and read about the role and responsibilities of personal tutors, as this may vary from university to university.

University services – student support and guidance

Outside of the student paramedics programme there will usually be a system of student support that has a university-wide focus. Services such as counselling, financial advice and student housing are commonly provided. Most universities have many more services; again, read the specific handbooks for your institution and you will find services and guidance that may be useful to you in the future. HEIs usually have strong support networks for their students and clear structures for accessing services.

Ambulance service support

During your periods of practice experience you will generally be supported by a registered paramedic who has additional experience and education to act as a mentor/PEd. If student paramedics are employed by the ambulance trust they may also be able to access the services offered for employed staff of the ambulance service. Again, more detailed information may be contained within the handbook that is specifically related to your institution and programme of study.

ᴄ⟩ Refer to Chapter 10 for more detail on all these roles.

This chapter has highlighted some of the ways in which studying for a paramedic qualification may be different from other subjects. The next chapter will explore more of what it means to be a professional and the expectations that come with the title *student paramedic*.

Suggested reading

Blaber, A.Y. and Harris, G. (2014) *Clinical Leadership for Paramedics.* Maidenhead: Open University Press.

Bolton, G.E.J. (2014) *Reflective Practice: Writing and Professional Development* (4th edn). London: Sage.

College of Paramedics (2014) *Paramedic Curriculum Guidance* (3rd edn). Bridgwater: College of Paramedics. Available at: https://www. collegeofparamedics.co.uk/downloads/Curriculum_Guidance_2014.pdf (accessed 18 February 2005).

Fleming, N.D. (2001) *Teaching and Learning Styles: VARK Strategies.* Christchurch, New Zealand: Neil Fleming.

Health and Care Professions Council (2014). *Standards of Education and Training.* London: HCPC. Available at: http://www.hcpc-uk.org.uk/ aboutregistration/standards/sets/index.asp (accessed 18 January 2015).

Honey, P. and Mumford, A. (1986) *Using your Learning Styles.* Maidenhead: Peter Honey.

Kolb, D. (1974) On management and the learning process. In D. Kolb, I. Rubin and J. McIntyre (eds) *Organizational Psychology* (2nd edn). Englewood Cliffs, NJ: Prentice Hall.

Richardson, M. (2012) Reflective practice in relation to pre-hospital care. In A.Y. Blaber (ed.) *Foundations for Paramedic Practice: A Theoretical Perspective* (2nd edn). Maidenhead: Open University Press.

Taylor, B.J. (2010) *Reflective Practice for Health Care Professionals: A Practical Guide* (3rd edn). Maidenhead: Open University Press.

Thompson, S. and Thompson, N. (2008) *The Critically Reflective Practitioner.* Basingstoke: Palgrave Macmillan.

4 WHAT IS A 'PROFESSIONAL' PROGRAMME?

Chapter 1 briefly mentioned the fact that paramedic studies incorporate both an academic and professional qualification. This means that you will leave your HEI with an academic qualification (diploma, foundation degree, BSc) and the eligibility to register with the HCPC at the point of successfully completing the period of study.

It has already been stated that health-care students are different than other university students, and the role of governing or professional bodies such as the Health and Care Professions Council (HCPC) and the College of Paramedics (CoP), and the impact they have on student paramedics, will be discussed further in this chapter. You will also have a chance to explore what constitutes professional behaviour as a paramedic – an important area that will impact on your final reference from your university to the HCPC.

What is the Health and Care Professions Council?

The HCPC is the regulatory body for paramedics. Many other allied health professions are also regulated by the HCPC – for example, physiotherapists and social workers. The main objective of the HCPC is to protect the public. There are four ways by which this is achieved (Clarke et al. 2012):

- the maintaining of a register of health professionals – including paramedics;
- the approval of education programmes leading to eligibility to apply for registration;
- the assessment of continuing professional development (CPD);
- the hearing of fitness to practise complaints.

The HCPC maintains the register of paramedics and only people whose names are on the register can use the title 'paramedic'. This is what is meant by a protected title. It is a criminal offence to use the title if your name does not appear on the HCPC register. The register is accessible online and anyone is able to cross-check a name or registration number.

The threshold requirements of the profession are detailed in the *Standards of Proficiency* for paramedics (HCPC 2014a), and the potential registrant must prove they have reached these, usually by successfully passing a programme of study that has been approved by the Education Committee of the HCPC. In addition to competence, the student paramedic must also have adhered to the *Guidance on Conduct and Ethics for Students* (HCPC 2012b) throughout their period of study.

Once on the register, the paramedic must be able to demonstrate their professional development by undertaking educational and professional study (CPD), develop a portfolio and adhere to the HCPC *Standards of Conduct, Performance and Ethics* (HCPC 2012a). Failure to achieve all of the above may – for a student – result in their failing their paramedic programme of study and not being eligible to register as a paramedic. For a registered paramedic, failure to adhere to the professional standards may result in a complaint, subsequent investigation, suspension from employment pending investigation, and, depending on the result of the hearing, ultimately removal from the register as a paramedic.

Box 4.1 refers to the role of the HCPC and provides guidance for students to undertake more investigation. The CoP is also mentioned and more detail is provided about this organisation in the section below.

Box 4.1 Comments about the role of the HCPC and CoP

🎓 **Academic response:** The HCPC is there to protect the public and ensure that its registrants maintain high personal and professional standards. In this way it endeavours to provide patients with the highest standard of care possible. It is good practice to start and maintain a portfolio early in your career, updating it as necessary. Templates for guidance are available on the HCPC website and give very good information. Many of the paramedics who fall foul of the HCPC and find themselves in trouble have been guilty of substandard paperwork. Make sure yours is always in order from day 1.

The College of Paramedics is influential in forming the future of paramedic education. It runs CPD events and produces the *Journal of Paramedic Practice* in which there are many interesting articles relevant to the profession. Whilst it is not a registering body, it does have influence.

Paramedic mentor/PEd response: Be aware at all times of how you come across to your patients and other members of the public. Do not cut corners either in practice or paperwork. These issues are some of the commonest causes of complaint to the HCPC, and being aware from the outset will hopefully avoid any problems.

It is worth joining the College of Paramedics in order to keep abreast of developments in our profession. It runs excellent CPD days and offers guidance and support to paramedics, both qualified and those still a student.

Student response: I know there are some countries where just about anybody can call themselves a paramedic after having had hardly any training or education. The fact that we have to register with a regulatory body which will only let us be called 'paramedics' once we have achieved a whole raft of criteria gives a value to the word 'paramedic' which is greater than anywhere else in the world – we're not just medics, we're HCPC paramedics! That means we have met a standard that the public can have confidence in and that we ourselves can have confidence in – the people who decide who can practise as paramedics have decided we are fit to practise, and that gives me a confidence I wouldn't have if I'd only done a first aid course and put on a green jumpsuit.

Paramedic/PEd response: It is important to understand your roles and responsibilities from day 1. Take time to explore the HCPC website – look through documents that it provides and understand how you will function individually. Likewise, review fitness to practise cases, familiarise yourself with the CPD guidance and learn how the HCPC functions in the development of the paramedic profession and educational programmes. Having an understanding and awareness of this will assist in your development from a general student to a professional student, and then into a health-care professional who takes great pride in obtaining and maintaining their registration and being part of a professional regulatory body. I would massively suggest becoming a member of the College of Paramedics early on; yes, there is a cost – but it is worth it! Lots of work goes into developing study days that are specifically aimed at the paramedic profession and delivered by specialists. Additionally, once you are registered there are CPD activities and guidance notes to help you continue your learning and development.

What is the College of Paramedics and what is its role?

The College of Paramedics is the recognised professional body for paramedics and the ambulance professions. Its main role is to 'represent ambulance professionals' in all matters affecting their clinical practice, and to 'provide support to the profession by providing advice to our members, and to people considering joining the ambulance professions' (CoP 2014b).

As with any professional body there is a membership cost, but this is significantly reduced for student paramedics, and with this membership comes access to numerous local CPD and educational events.

Another aspect of the CoP's work is to support HEIs in development of programmes of study. All programmes on the UCAS website have been through internal scrutiny by the individual university's quality processes and external scrutiny from the HCPC before finally gaining validation by the HCPC. This process can take up to a year or more to achieve from inception to successful validation. Curriculum guidance from the CoP (2014a: 19) details the approval and endorsement of programmes:

> In 2012 the College of Paramedics launched its own endorsement scheme, which provided a further layer of quality assurance for users and providers of educational programmes, over and above existing standards set by the HCPC and QAA [Quality Assurance Agency] ... endorsement will only be awarded to pre-registration programmes at academic level 6 in England, Wales and Northern Ireland and, in Scotland, the Scottish Bachelors degree SHE level 3 (SCQF9) from the academic year 2015/16.

So you may also see the CoP logo on university presentations/paperwork. This denotes that the programme you are investigating has been through the CoP endorsement process, in addition to the HCPC and internal university validation.

Having discussed some aspects of academic study in Chapter 3, it is appropriate to examine what is meant by the term *professional behaviour*.

Professional behaviour

The HCPC (2012b) guidance on conduct and ethics for students makes clear that any concern relating to conduct or, more accurately, misconduct, outside your programme of study is important and that there are certain professional responsibilities. It is clear that conduct outside of study is scrutinised and in serious circumstances may affect the student's ability to complete their studies, gain the final qualification or register with the HCPC. Some definitions of professional behaviour are given in Box 4.2.

Box 4.2 How would you define the term *professional behaviour*?

🎓 **Academic response:** Professional behaviour can be defined as conforming to the technical or ethical standards of one's profession. For many health professions, including paramedics, these standards are explicitly set out by the HCPC. Some are generic and some profession-specific. These standards should be adhered to all the time and do not become of less value just because you may be having a bad shift.

🗼 **Paramedic mentor/PEd response:** It is important to understand that professional behaviour applies not only when you are at work but also in your personal life. Take care when using social media. Many students and qualified paramedics have posted 'inappropriate' information which may be indefensible if questioned.

🗼 **Paramedic mentor/PEd response:** For me this is quite simply the most important thing. I view professional behaviour as a multitude of actions and not just the way that you conduct yourself at work. You wear a uniform, so wearing this smartly and with pride to represent your profession, the language you choose to use daily, the actions you choose to take outside of work that impact on the public's perception of you (you never know when that person may just be your patient) and the way you conduct yourself in work, with colleagues and patients alike – all go towards developing your professional behaviour. How you behave at university and in your private life is equally important because, speaking from experience, you get noticed there as well. Social media – well, all I would say is use it appropriately. Professional behaviour overall, for me, is who you are, we have all chosen a profession that makes us hugely recognisable in the public eye, and we will be noticed. Remembering that, both inside and outside of work, doesn't stop you from having fun and enjoying your journey, but it does stop you from simply getting into a whole world of problems.

📖 **Student paramedic response:** The public often don't know you are a student. We wear the uniform of our ambulance trust. So you are dressed in the same green uniform as paramedics with advanced clinical skills, it's only your epaulettes/name badge which mark out the difference. You are representing a lot of other people when you put that uniform on, not just yourself. The public see the ambulance service as a whole and other paramedics get an impression of your university when they look at you and the way you behave. Act like a professional even before you become one.

Being professional, in my opinion, means being the best paramedic you can be and doing the best you can do for your patient. It's treating every patient like they are a relative of yours. If your mum needed a paramedic today, how would you want her to be treated? The elderly lady you get called out to is someone's mum or gran. Treat them like your own.

The HCPC (2012b: 9–12) provides 13 main points of guidance on conduct and ethics for students, with further detail provided on each point. Take time to read through Table 4.1 carefully and refer to the HCPC document itself for more detail.

Some of the terminology used in Table 4.1 may not be familiar to you and will require further reading, such as informed consent. Do not worry too much about this, as your programme of study will address these concepts in more detail and relate them to the work of a paramedic.

Good character

On successfully completing an educational programme of study the student paramedic will be asked for information as part of a declaration of *good character* and this forms one part of the application process to join the HCPC register as a paramedic. This includes declaring the following:

- any convictions or cautions;
- being disciplined by a professional organisation, regulator or employer; or
- having any civil proceedings made against you.

Table 4.1 Guidance on conduct and ethics for students

You should always act in the best interests of your service users.
You should respect the confidentiality of your service users.
You should keep high standards of personal conduct.
You should provide any important information about your conduct, competence or health to your education provider.
You should limit your study or stop studying if your performance or judgement is affected by your health.
You should keep your professional knowledge and skills up to date.
You should act within the limits of your knowledge and skills.
You should communicate effectively with service users and your education provider and placement providers.
You should get informed consent to provide care or service (so far as possible).
You should keep accurate records on service users.
You should deal fairly and safely with the risks of infection.
You should behave honestly.
You should make sure that your behaviour does not damage public confidence in your profession.

It is clear that any misconduct outside (or as part of) the programme of study is a serious matter and may affect your long-term career aspirations. In this sense you should not see your behaviour and conduct inside and outside the university/placement area as being separate. Your conduct at all times needs to be of a high standard and appropriate to a professional who will be eligible to apply for the protected title of paramedic.

The next few subsections are intended to draw your attention to areas where there are high expectations for student paramedics.

Attitude

Conduct includes one's attitude to colleagues, service users, families and academic/practice staff. The HCPC (2012b) expects the student to be polite and to communicate appropriately and effectively with service users, colleagues, academic and placement teams. Inappropriate attitudes to any parties can potentially be construed as misconduct. Some advice is given in Box 4.3.

⌀ Refer to Chapter 1 and the discussion about communication and its importance in health-care environments.

Box 4.3 What is your advice to students about their attitude?

🎓 **Academic response:** Your attitude can have a massive effect on the effectiveness of your interactions with patients, carers, fellow students and tutors alike. A negative attitude can easily be detected in your body language. At best this will impede your communication, at worst it may result in complaints or escalate potentially violent situations.

🚑 **Paramedic mentor/PEd response:** Attitude is so important. Remember that people who call for an ambulance are often frightened and in pain. What may seem minor to you may be the end of the world to them. We are not in a position to judge our patients – we do not know the road that led them to where they are now. Treat all patients with respect and dignity. Putting a patient at ease will often change an obstructive attitude to one of cooperation. It is very rare that I have been unable to talk round even the most aggressive patient by maintaining a non-judgemental and friendly attitude.

🎓 **Academic response:** The HCPC provides advice to students in its *Guidance on Conduct and Ethics for Students*. Students are required to conduct themselves in line with this guidance and can find themselves in serious trouble if they do not, which can lead to fitness to practise processes within their HEI being initiated.

📖 **Student response:** When you think about it we are a service industry aiming to give 'customer satisfaction'. OK, we don't call our service users 'customers', but the principle is there. We want people who use the service to have a positive experience of it even when, sadly, the outcome of their call is not a happy one. A caring and professional attitude goes without saying, but I learnt that you can never underestimate the way in which having this attitude can help calm people, or benefit a situation.

People who have had to call an ambulance often say 'the paramedics were brilliant'. You then find out that they are referring to an event from years ago – people never forget what you have done for them or how you acted; even if it was just another job to you, it could well have been a defining moment for them. Our attitude at work can generate letters from the public, both good and bad. I prefer the good ones!

🎓 **Academic response:** It is important to remember that attitude extends to your time in university and the various placements you will undertake as well as your time on shift. Being polite and treating others with respect is imperative. The adage 'manners cost nothing' is very true. You can 'ace' your academic work and still be marked down on your conduct and attitude. This subjective area is probably one of the most important in paramedic practice. Ask yourself often, 'how do you come across to others?'

It is clear from the comments in Box 4.3 that attitude encompasses both practice and academic areas of your life and will affect your relationships.

Timekeeping and appearance

Part of professional behaviour is your timekeeping and appearance. Many students are under the misapprehension that timekeeping when in university is less important than when reporting for shifts with their mentors. Both practice and academic staff are noting lateness; in some institutions registers are taken and lateness officially recorded. Any academic asked to write a reference for a student at the end of their studies may be asked by the employer to record episodes of lateness/sickness and absence. It is their professional duty (your lecturers are also professionals with registrations to professional regulatory bodies) to report this as accurately and honestly as possible. So the student's performance and professional conduct is under scrutiny in both the academic and practice environment.

When in the practice environment students are required to adhere to the uniform policy for their ambulance trust or, if not provided with a uniform, the clothes policy for the programme provided by the university (for the purposes of this chapter the term 'uniform' will be used). Some university study may require students to wear their uniforms in the classroom or simulation environment. Students need to be aware that on such occasions full uniform should be worn and appearance should be as smart as when on placement.

You are invited into people's homes, and you are the first point of contact many of your patients will have with the NHS. Your attitude and appearance are what people will use to make their first judgement. It is important to make an excellent first impression, as the comments in Box 4.4 highlight. If you needed a paramedic, who would you rather have care for you: a smart, friendly, helpful paramedic, or one who looks dishevelled, wearing an unironed uniform and dirty boots, who looks unenthusiastic and is unfriendly?

Box 4.4 What do you believe is the value (or not) of your uniform?

📖 **Student paramedic response:** When you first get your uniform it is tempting to be seen wearing it. We were warned about not going 'clubbing' in it or wearing it down the high street when popping out for some milk! Sometimes, though, when you're on your way to the start of your shift and have to stop to get petrol or nip into the supermarket to get your meal deal for lunch you may be in uniform. I always put a coat over my uniform in that situation so all people could see was my green trousers – then I looked as much like a landscape gardener as anything else! I didn't want to stroll into Sainsbury's looking like a paramedic when I wasn't yet one. Supposing someone collapsed in the 'seasonal goods' aisle – everyone would expect me to leap in and do something! Being in uniform outside of your shift is false advertising! Why put yourself in that situation?

🚨 **Paramedic mentor/PEd response:** Appearance is important! Be proud of the uniform you wear. It may be Christmas, but will the family of the patient in cardiac arrest really be filled with optimism when they see the flashing Santa badge pinned to your lapel or the tinsel taking the place of your bootlaces?

🚨 **Paramedic mentor/PEd response:** I think uniform has high regard and value with the job we do and serves a purpose. First and foremost, it encourages a professional attitude, as we display the crest and badge of the service for whom we work. Secondly, it sends the message that everyone is equal within the organisation, as for the lay person we are all in the same uniform. We wear epaulettes that provide distinction of grade.

Practically, it is tough, can be washed over and over, and is designed to minimise injury to you through its simple ergonomic design.

🎓 **Academic response:** First impressions count! Patients will be far more willing to trust and cooperate with a smart, friendly paramedic than one who slouches into the job with shirt tails hanging, upset at being called out in the early hours.

Sickness and absence

Students should make sure they are aware of the procedures to report in sick to both academic institutions and practice areas. This information is usually available from programme handbooks.

The number of hours accrued in the practice environment is specific to individual programmes, but the HCPC sets a minimum amount of hours required in order to be eligible to register. Hence the importance of recording hours in both theory and practice.

Students should keep their own record of sickness and absence; official university and practice records can sometimes not reflect what either party believe to be accurate. This is important information and will be requested by potential employers when you are applying for jobs.

Consent

The term *consent* means obtaining the person's permission. For paramedics it usually refers to permission to do something to them, such as taking blood pressure. In health care the term *informed consent* is often used and is referred to in Table 4.1. The HCPC (2012a: 11) defines informed consent as follows: 'when someone has all the information they need, in a format they can understand, to make a decision about receiving care or services'. I would also suggest that it could also be about the person's decision *not to* receive care or services. Box 4.5 contains some examples of situations where consent may be difficult to obtain.

Box 4.5 An example of when informed consent may be difficult to obtain

🚨 **Paramedic response:** Wherever possible, gain consent from your patient and explain to them what is happening. In some cases this may be impossible, for example, unconscious patients or those with lowered levels of consciousness. This should not be a problem as long as you are working in the best interests of the patient at *all* times.

🚨 **Paramedic response:** Obtaining informed consent is difficult when there are significant language barriers, especially when there is no one available to translate. Whilst there is the option to utilise language lines (which I recommend), where translation can happen over the phone, in this situation you could initiate a process by physically demonstrating what is required and sending and receiving communication gestures.

🎓 **Academic response:** Consent need not be explicit. Implied consent is just as valid as that which is explicitly given. An example of this is, if you ask a patient permission to cannulate and they offer you their arm. Keep your patients informed of what is happening at all times. They have a right to know in order that they can make an informed judgement. Talking and reassurance pay dividends.

📖 **Student paramedic response:** Consent is not just a one-off thing you ask for at the start of your assessment; it can be situation-specific at times. For example, just because I have been given permission to take my patient's blood pressure, I don't assume they have given consent for me to start unbuttoning their top and attach the 12 lead stickers! I will tell the patient what assessment observations I need to take and what the procedure involves in a way they can appreciate, and ask 'is that OK?' before proceeding. Often they will pre-empt me and offer their arm for the blood pressure cuff or their finger to take a sample of blood to measure their blood sugar, which is implied consent. Even if they say 'do whatever you need to do', I will still inform them before doing anything, just in case they meant 'do whatever you need to do – except the procedure you're about to'.

> **Reflection: point to consider**
>
> Think about the potential issues with gaining consent for someone who is unconscious. What do you think are the issues here?

Consent is a concept that needs to be continually in your mind, and you may need to adapt your practice accordingly. You will meet various situations, as described in Box 4.5, and many will require discussion with your mentor/PEd. You are learning – when in doubt, ask, and do some investigation for yourself.

> **CASE STUDY 4.1**
>
> Attending patients who are under the influence of alcohol can provide a multitude of issues in relation to obtaining informed consent – assuming that the patient is conscious, behaviour will vary individually. Some people will find the situation they are in highly amusing, others will be sad, some aggressive, and it is vital to ensure that you have their attention and that any information you give them is appropriately understood and that you are able to get a reply that you believe shows their understanding. This is easier said than done. The difficulty is that the longer you take trying to get this consent the longer it is taking to obtain these interventions. It is important to remember that you are working in the best interest of the patient.

Case Study 4.1 highlights the potential difficulty and volatility when caring for patients under the influence of alcohol. The value of excellent communication skills cannot be emphasised enough.

Consent is complex and is an integral part of any student paramedic programme, so the legal and ethical issues surrounding informed consent will be addressed during your studies.

Confidentiality

Confidentiality refers to both practice and academic work. Information about service users that was given to you in the line of your work as a student paramedic is confidential. It should only be used 'for the purpose for which it was given, unless the information raises concerns about a situation where someone may be at risk' (HCPC 2012a: 19).

As a student, you should not pass on any details about a service user without the permission of your mentor/PEd. When in doubt, check, or err on the side of caution.

Student paramedic comment: Patients trust us with information about themselves and their health which they may not want shared with other people. It's obvious that we would never deliberately break this confidentiality, but I have heard of occasions where paramedics have been in situations where confidentiality could be compromised. You never know whether the member of the public who is in earshot of your conversation about a patient with another paramedic is not actually a relative of that patient – you could unknowingly let out some information the relative didn't know which significantly alters their relationship to the patient (not good!).

It is important to note that confidentiality is not always broken maliciously, as Case Study 4.2 demonstrates.

CASE STUDY 4.2 EXAMPLE OF CONFIDENTIALITY IN DIFFERING CIRCUMSTANCES

A paramedic was working on a rapid response vehicle and was using paper patient report forms. After finishing a job she would place the patient report forms on the 'dash' of the vehicle. These had been placed face up with patient information visible. On returning to station for a break an officer saw the patient records and was able to read confidential information.

It appears that the paramedic imagined that the physical barrier of the windscreen would keep the patient information safe and that others would not make a point of reading information from the clipboard. A simple mistake and lack of appreciation of the wider meaning of confidentiality led to a breach of patient confidentiality for the patient and quite serious consequences for the paramedic, in the form of disciplinary action.

Sally, in Case Study 4.3, fully understands her professional responsibilities both during and outside of work situations. A less experienced or less well informed paramedic than Sally may have experienced difficulties in a similar situation. It is important to understand confidentiality in all its guises and in a variety of situations in order to appreciate the complexity of situations that you may find yourself in.

CASE STUDY 4.3 EXAMPLE OF CONFIDENTIALITY IN DIFFERING CIRCUMSTANCES

A paramedic (Sally) was asked for advice by a friend (Bob). Bob's partner had problems and needed to speak to someone. Sally did not know Bob's partner but agreed to speak to her on the telephone to see if she could advise her. It must be stressed here that this was in Sally's own time and not in work time. When Sally spoke to Bob's partner it became apparent from her medication that she had a history of severe mental health problems and psychotic episodes. It was obvious that Bob was not aware of this. When Bob asked Sally what the matter was and if she had been able to help, Sally could not comment. To do so would have been a blatant breach of confidentiality. Remember that confidentiality issues do not go away just because you are out of work and not on shift.

It is important that you clearly understand your institution's policies regarding confidentiality when writing assignments and examinations. Read and clarify the policy with your lecturers, as this may vary from institution to institution.

Confidentiality and social networking sites are inextricably linked, yet many students need the link to be made clear to them.

Social networking sites

Reflection: points to consider

Think about the last five things you posted on Facebook or any other social networking forum.

Do you think you would be happy for your university lecturers to see what you posted?

What does the content of your page say about you?

What impressions might an outsider form of you, without meeting you, from looking at your posts?

The HCPC has amended its student guidance on conduct and ethics to include the use of social media (HCPC 2012a). It is an area that many registrants and students find lacks clarity. The first point is that information placed on these sites is in the public domain and can therefore be viewed by other people. Even if it is on a private group/page, it is classified as being viewable by anyone, and you do not know who is accessing others computers.

The HCPC (2012a) document, which you should read in full, says:

> When you post information on social networking sites, think about whether it is appropriate to share that information. If the information is confidential and is about your service user, patient, client or colleague, you should not put it on a site. This could include information about their personal life, health or circumstances.

You do not need to include their name in order to break confidentiality. The document warns:

> we might need to take action if the comments posted were offensive, for example if they were racist or sexually explicit.

In short, do not enter into any social networking discussion that involves patient care or comments relating to anyone you have cared for, colleagues, academics or friends, for that matter. The advice given in Box 4.6 reiterates the importance of understanding the potential consequences of your actions when engaged with social media.

Box 4.6 Advice on social media use for student paramedics

🎓 **Academic response:** Go to the HCPC website, click the 'complaints' tab and then take a look at the 'hearings' section to see reasons why registrants (not necessarily just paramedics) have been disciplined or struck off. Too many of them are related to inappropriate use of social media. Such a waste of a career!

🚨 **Paramedic mentor/PEd response:** Be very, very careful how you use social media. What will your trust think about photographs of you in uniform? Think twice about the posts you share, the language you use and the opinions you voice. Many staff have ended up in serious trouble because of the thoughtless use of social media.

🚨 **Paramedic response:** A moment's madness on a social networking site could cause a lifetime of sadness if it costs you your career.

📖 **Student paramedic response:** We were warned that photos on Facebook of us in uniform and/or in a compromising situation were an absolute no-no. Also, putting up things about jobs we'd been to which could potentially breach confidentiality were an obvious thing to avoid. I guess the rule is: don't put up anything you wouldn't be happy for your programme leader, paramedic mentor or work colleagues to see.

🎓 **Academic response:** Many more employers are implementing social media searches of prospective employees, to judge professionalism and suitability for employment. Carry on using social media in an unprofessional way and you may not even get to this point. HEIs and ambulance partners will not tolerate inappropriate use by student paramedics.

What about you personally, then, posting photographs of yourself in uniform, for instance? The HCPC (2012a) says: 'You must behave with honesty and integrity and make sure that your behaviour does not damage the public's confidence in you or your profession.'

It could be argued that a photograph of you standing in your uniform is innocuous enough, but who is to say that the photograph will not be used by someone else, altered and then appear elsewhere as an inappropriate and unprofessional image? Ultimately it is your responsibility for posting it initially. Please check your individual university and practice area policies on social media usage for specific details relating to your localities.

It is hoped that this chapter has raised your awareness of some important issues related to becoming a professional. Sometimes students can make innocent mistakes, but the key is to be honest, act with integrity and learn from your mistakes (and those of others) during the course of your studies and experiences in clinical practice.

Suggested reading

Clarke, V., Harris, G. and Cowland, S. (2012) Ethics and law for the paramedic. In A.Y. Blaber (ed.) *Foundations for Paramedic Practice: A Theoretical Perspective* (2nd edn). Maidenhead: Open University Press.

College of Paramedics (2014) *Paramedic Curriculum Guidance* (3rd edn). Bridgwater: College of Paramedics. Available at: https://www.collegeofparamedics.co.uk/downloads/Curriculum_Guidance_2014.pdf (accessed 18 February 2005).

College of Paramedics (2014b) *College of Paramedics. About us.* Available at: https://www.collegeofparamedics.co.uk/about_us/welcome (accessed 18 January 2015).

Harris, G. and Fellows, R. (2012) Continuing professional development: pre and post registration. In A.Y. Blaber (ed.) *Foundations for Paramedic Practice: A Theoretical Perspective* (2nd edn). Maidenhead: Open University Press.

Health and Care Professions Council (2012a) *Standards of Conduct, Performance and Ethics.* London: HCPC. Available at: http://www.hcpc-uk.org/assets/documents/10003B6EStandardsofconduct,performanceandethics.pdf (accessed 18 January 2015).

Health and Care Professions Council (2012b) *Guidance on Conduct and Ethics for Students.* London: HCPC. Available at: http://www.hcpc-uk.org/assets/documents/10002C16Guidanceonconductandethicsforstudents.pdf (accessed 18 January 2015).

Health and Care Professions Council (2014a) *Standards of Proficiency. Paramedics.* London: HCPC. Available at: http://www.hpc-uk.org/assets/

documents/1000051CStandards_of_Proficiency_Paramedics.pdf (accessed 18 January 2015).

Health and Care Professions Council (2014b) *Focus on Standards – Social Networking Sites*. London: HCPC. Available at: www.hcpc-uk.org/Assets/documents/1003587Social_medica_guidance.pdf (accessed 18 January 2015).

5   WHAT WILL I BE STUDYING?

Your studies to become a paramedic will be as complex as the needs of your patients. You need to understand the whole patient in order to be able to care for them safely and effectively. This concept is known as *holistic* care. The subjects you will be learning about are diverse in order to prepare you to care for your patients in a holistic way.

Reflection: points to consider

List the academic subjects you think will help you to understand most things about your patient.

List the academic subjects you do not think will be useful to you and your patients.

The HCPC (2014b) *Standards of Education and Training* (SETs) set out the duties of the education provider. This is one aspect that the HCPC measures any programme against before an institution can offer a paramedic programme to students. The SETs cover six broad areas, as seen in Table 5.1.

In addition to the very broad SETs described in Table 5.1, the education provider uses the *Standards of Proficiency* (HCPC 2014a) and the College of Paramedics (2014) *Curriculum Guidance* document to develop a programme that meets the governing and professional bodies' exacting standards and will provide the student with eligibility to register on successful completion. It is these documents that provide clear direction on the subjects that require inclusion in any paramedic programme.

What subjects will I be studying?

The curriculum content recommended by the College of Paramedics is listed in Table 5.2, and the proficiencies required by the registrant (HCPC 2014a) are listed in Table 5.3. Bear in mind that Table 5.2 only lists the

Table 5.1 Areas covered by the HCPC (2014b) *Standards of Education and Training* (SETS)

1. Level of qualification for entry to the register

2. Programme admissions

3. Programme management and resources

4. Curriculum

5. Practice placements

6. Assessment

Table 5.2 College of Paramedics (2014) curriculum content categories

Physical sciences, e.g. gases, acids, bases, diffusion

Life sciences, e.g. study of major body systems and associated physiology (normal and altered)

Social, health and behavioural sciences, e.g. sociology, psychology, social policy

Clinical sciences, e.g. lifespan and altered physiology and illnesses, pharmacology

Ethics and law and professional issues that inform and shape paramedic practice

Patient assessment

Care delivery, e.g. theoretical and practical skills that are required when providing care

Leadership attributes

Evidence- and research-based practice

broad categories of the topics of study; the full guidance document provides much more detail.

Any paramedic programme is much more than a skills-based qualification, something that comes as a surprise to many students. You may be familiar with some of the categories. Or you may be surprised by some of the subjects that are included, such as leadership and research. It is important to mention that your university team do not expect you to have studied all of these subjects before commencing the programme. There is a wide range of subjects to be studied and some subject areas may be completely new to you.

In your cohort you will have a mixture of colleagues, some with more of a science background, others who prefer the social sciences – this is usual! Diversity in your cohort is healthy, and it also generally means you are able to learn from each other, in respect of academic subject content but also utilising your own experiences.

Table 5.3 HCPC (2014a) *Standards of Proficiency* for paramedics

Registrant paramedics must:
1 be able to practise safely and effectively within their scope of practice
2 be able to practise within the legal and ethical boundaries of their profession
3 be able to maintain fitness to practise
4 be able to practise as an autonomous professional, exercising their own professional judgement
5 be aware of the impact of culture, equality and diversity on practice
6 be able to practise in a non-discriminatory manner
7 understand the importance of and be able to maintain confidentiality
8 be able to communicate effectively
9 be able to work appropriately with others
10 be able to maintain records appropriately
11 be able to reflect on and review practice
12 be able to assure the quality of their practice
13 understand the key concepts of the knowledge base relevant to their profession
14 be able to draw on appropriate knowledge and skills to inform practice
15 understand the need to establish and maintain a safe practice environment

As with the College of Paramedics document, the HCPC *Standards of Proficiency* listed in Table 5.3 also have explanatory notes if you look at the whole document.

You can see that the two documents referred to in Tables 5.2 and 5.3 interact and complement one another.

Table 5.3 shows that, in addition to clearly defined subjects on the course, such as anatomy and physiology, there are other professional aspects that are equally as important, for example non-discriminatory practice and maintaining records.

Do all programmes cover similar content?

The general answer to this is yes. Institutions will have developed their para-medic curricula based around the HCPC SETs, *Standards of Proficiency* and College of Paramedics (2014) curriculum guidance. There will be some variation on where in the programme the students receive some content. For example, some programmes may decide that patient assessment needs to be taught at the end of year 1, for others it will be in year 2. Some of this decision-making may result from the partnership arrangement with the ambulance service. This will result in a joint decision between the HEI and ambulance trust about what clinical skills will be taught and at what point in the programme it is most appropriate. This will vary from area to area of the UK and from programme to programme. Whatever the case, you can be assured that your programme has been scrutinised by internal university quality processes and the HCPC, as a minimum requirement.

Some of the areas you cover during lectures may be on the brief side. With such a wide range of subjects to cover, academic teams have to decide what subjects will be covered in most detail and what others can be learned via other learning and teaching methods, such as independent and guided study, workshops and simulation. In some situations there may be guided study provided as a way of extending your knowledge further and exceeding the academic level you need. Clear guidance will be given on this and it is then up to you, as the adult learner, to choose to complete it or not.

Student paramedic comment: The programme I did covered a range of subjects from anatomy to sociology. At first some students questioned the relevance of some topics – why learn about sociology? Once they'd been out on placement and saw how sociology is relevant to the way people live, the situations they get into and how this impacts upon us as paramedics they realised how useful these subjects are and that the programme had been carefully structured.

I'd also say that at university we weren't just training to do a job, we were studying a subject – paramedic science/practice. As a result we gained a far wider and deeper understanding of the paramedic role, not just knowledge of how to cannulate. I feel this gave us the foundation for greater development personally and professionally. Uni is not simply about training, it's about education.

The wide range of subject areas is one major reason why independent study is essential to your success.

What is independent study?

This may be called different things in different institutions – for example, self-directed study or study time. Independent study is entirely in the hands of the student. Your academic staff can suggest periods of independent study by allocating time during a module/unit; this usually will appear on a timetable. Guided study usually has set reading or a set task or work that needs to be completed and taken to the next lecture. It is different from independent study, where what you do with your time is entirely up to you, as Box 5.1 illustrates.

Box 5.1 Do students use independent study?

🎓 **Academic response:** This is really down to the individual and is often directly proportional to a student's prior experience of higher education. Many students who have not experienced university learning before expect everything to be 'spoon-fed' in class. I always say that in university you are 'treated as a grown-up' and we expect you to delve further into subjects we only have time to introduce you to in class. It will be useful for you to ask your tutors to give you broad areas for self-study.

🚑 **Paramedic mentor/PEd response:** The more driven the student, the more time I find they devote to self-study. It is the students who really want to be paramedics that tend to go the extra mile with their studies.

🚑 **Paramedic mentor/PEd response:** Independent study varies massively depending on the student's enthusiasm and willingness to learn. No matter what the structure of the student's programme of study is, the willingness to learn while on practice varies from student to student. A student who wants to know as much as possible is always looking to broaden their knowledge on things they have seen on placement and will spend their time doing this. Students may spend time before placements researching areas they want to discuss and develop with their mentors. Unfortunately, some students think that the knowledge they need is purely based on

---

what is taught as part of their programme and view independent study as a day off. My advice would be to use independent study time to the best of your ability; you will never know enough.

📖 **Student paramedic response:** My motivation for independent study consisted of equal parts of fascination and fear. I investigated a subject to a deeper level outside of lectures often because I was fascinated by it and had a hunger to learn more, but also because I was dead scared of not knowing enough and failing an exam or essay. This approach may not have been ideal, but it paid off. I got some good grades and a better level of understanding on many subjects than I would have without it.

On some programmes there are set weeks of independent study, on others there are individual days. However your programme is organised, there will be some dedicated time allocated for you to study. Other study will be required on your days off, especially as deadlines approach. But remember you are studying for life, not just to pass modules/units. All of the information you will be gathering is useful for your career development and much of it will be used on a daily basis, not simply learnt for an examination and then never used again!

Generally the most effective way of really learning something is to learn it over a period of time, review it periodically and use your knowledge in practice regularly. This is why academics will advocate reading regularly and not just cramming for deadlines, as this is the material that you forget once the deadline has passed. Cramming may not make you the best paramedic that you can be and you may not realise your potential by using the cramming approach to studies. Being challenged in practice (in a friendly and supportive way) is an excellent way to recall what you know (or have forgotten) and to link theory to practice. I would suggest that any patient that you meet in practice would be useful to write up about consciously for your independent study. An example of this is found in Case Study 5.1.

CASE STUDY 5.1

Lily is 75 years old. She lives with her husband and she has a long-term history of emphysema. Lily has home oxygen and regularly takes her peak flow reading. She is on numerous medications and really does not like being hospitalised. She has called 999 as her peak flow measurements are lower than normal. Five days ago, Lily was diagnosed by her GP as having a chest infection. Lily has been taking the antibiotics prescribed by her GP for 4 days now.

Your independent study could be structured in the following ways:

● Understanding the anatomy and physiology of the normal respiratory system.
● Understanding the altered physiology of emphysema and how common it is.
● What is the treatment and management for people with emphysema?
● What are the likely medications Lily would be on and what doses, and how do they work?
● What is a peak flow, what is normal, and what does a change indicate? Are there any local/national guidelines on this?
● How do you document your findings and action?
● How do you assess Lily physically, psychologically and socially?
● Why might Lily not like being in hospital?
● What might be the effect of living with a debilitating long-term condition for someone of her age?
● What help is there that you may be able to access?
● What would you do if Lily refused to go to hospital? What are your responsibilities, ethically and legally?
● Could the care you gave to Lily been improved? Does the knowledge that you now have mean you would alter her care in any way, and would you do anything differently? On reflection, what have you learnt?

As you can see from Case Study 5.1, you do not have much information about Lily in the above scenario, yet there are so many questions that can be asked about each patient interaction that you have. These can be examined in as much or as little depth as you individually want, depending on how inquisitive you naturally are and how much you make an attempt to critically analyse. It is pertinent to mention the issue of consent when writing about patients in academic work. You will be required to gain consent and maintain confidentiality not only for the purpose of providing treatment but also when writing about patients in your academic work. The policies regarding consent and confidentiality for academic work vary from institution to institution, so you need to be clear what they are before including details of cases in your work. Falling foul of these rules can lead in some cases to a zero mark.

Using your patients to help you study independently is really useful, makes your learning pertinent and real, and most students seem to think this approach is a useful and effective one. Of course, there will be occasions when this approach will need to be supplemented by pure theory and it may not suit all types of learners.

🔗 Refer to the discussion on learning styles in Chapter 3.

What is guided study?

The term 'guided study' can be used to describe a variety of study methods. Guided study is generally a means of helping the student to focus their attention to a specific area or subject. This can be achieved by asking the student to complete work before a given lecture takes place. Lecturers will generally not cover this material again; they will assume the student has completed the guided study, as referred to in Box 5.2. If your lecturer

---

Box 5.2 How useful, or not, did you find guided study material?

🚨 **Paramedic response:** Whilst studying for my paramedic degree, I used quite a lot of guided study, particularly in my first year. I felt it was important to use my spare time wisely to prepare myself for the further two years, which became much busier. It was really helpful that our tutors did this for us as it gave a framework rather than staring blankly at a textbook and not knowing where to begin. Using guided study stood me in good stead for my career; now I'm registered I use a similar framework with any CPD I do, keeping my knowledge and practice up to date.

🚨 **Paramedic mentor/PEd response:** To support the use of guided study in university, as a mentor I adopt the following approaches with my students. I initially advise students to highlight any areas of practice they feel they personally need to learn and develop in and suggest independent study, which we can then discuss at a later date and use a question-and-answer session to test understanding. To encourage reflection and self-learning I encourage students to keep a record of incidents we attend and advise they do further literature searches and critical reads which I see and we can spend time discussing. I also find out what the student is currently studying at university. I can then, across the course of a number of shifts, focus our discussions, learning opportunities and the student's involvement in cases that are relevant to their stage of study. Letting the mentor have a copy of your timetable so that they know what you are studying allows them to facilitate situations where you can demonstrate your learning and understanding with a real patient, thus fulfilling your potential. I encourage students to be adequately prepared and bring appropriate resources to placements, such as reference books, a realistic plan of what they want to achieve and how they wish to achieve it and a positive attitude to wanting to learn. I like to develop a two-way working process with students, and encourage that as much as I can to help students learn and progress. There is knowledge that you have learnt at university, and a good way of consolidating this is to teach it to me!

PEd response: Knowing where to direct your study is extremely helpful for a number of reasons. It helps to break down masses of information into bite-sized pieces which stops students from feeling overwhelmed. It can save a lot of wasted time, particularly regarding exam revision. There is nothing more soul-destroying than spending hours revising a particular area only to find that you have concentrated on the wrong things.

Academic response: Guided study material is not an extra, it is key to the content I will deliver in a lecture. Students are directed to read/complete the guided study before attending the lecture; this will form the basis of the information required prior to the lecture and will usually be quite basic in nature. I will not revisit this information in the lecture. I can then concentrate on the more complex aspects of the subject, discuss them and answer any questions the group may have. Students who do not complete the guided study are at a significant disadvantage.

takes this approach, you may be somewhat lost in the lecture if you have not completed the guided study, as the work you should have done would have prepared you for the lecture content.

As you can see from the responses from the mentors/PEds in Box 5.2, guided study is not just a university-based approach. Some mentors/ PEds are extremely proactive and embrace a clearly structured teaching role whilst spending time with their student. This will help to bring the theory to life for the student and affords some excellent learning opportunities. Some guided study can be additional to the university lecture and module/unit content. It may be made up of a series of worksheets/workbooks that supplement the taught content and help you to appreciate the points made in the lecture, as the other comments in Box 5.2 highlight.

Learning support needs

Many students have individual learning support needs that will have been assessed at their school/college, and they have the support they require individually detailed for them. If you have declared this on your UCAS form, the HEI will usually have contacted you prior to commencing your studies to discuss your individual requirements and arrangements. All institutions have dedicated staff to assist both student and academics in providing the correct support, as Box 5.3 discusses. Be aware that the way this is managed may be different from what you have experienced to date, so it would be wise to find out how the system in your university works.

If you know you will need learning support it would be wise to ensure your lecturers know about it. As you commence your paramedic programme it may be worth mentioning it to your lecturers, or at least your programme leader or personal tutor. This will enable them to check what has been agreed for you individually, and that it is facilitated for you throughout your studies.

Additionally, some students experience difficulty with studying while at university and their lecturers may advise them to seek support, and this may lead to an assessment of individual learning needs. A student will generally be supported through this process by a person who usually has more experience than your lecturers in this area.

Box 5.3 What kinds of learning support needs do your colleagues have?

:🚨: **PEd response:** A surprisingly large number of students (and qualified paramedics returning to study) have additional learning support needs, so the first thing to emphasise is that you should not feel embarrassed to ask for support. This may feel like a big deal to you, but it is certainly no big deal to academic staff or colleagues. Additional support can be something as simple as having learning materials made available early, being able to record lectures or having extra reading time in exams. Don't suffer in silence! Support is very easy to arrange and may make a huge difference to the success of your studies.

🎓 **Academic response:** Students who arrive at university with a learning support need are identified early on and receive assessment and support before the term commences. The system is structured and generally works well. Sometimes students will discuss difficulties with their personal tutor, and we can then work with the student to get appropriate assessment, help and support – some issues may have been overlooked or missed at school or college. It is good for the student to finally be able to achieve their potential and realise there is a bona-fide reason for their difficulties; it is often a relief for the student and their confidence is boosted.

As Box 5.3 describes many students are in this situation. Do not worry about discussing this with staff at your university: they will know how to help you or put you in touch with someone who has the necessary expertise.

This chapter has explained what you can expect from your paramedic studies and how you will be studying a broad range of subjects. It is hoped that some useful suggestions have been made to help you understand why studying independently across the course of the year is important and how you can best do this effectively.

Suggested reading/websites

College of Paramedics (2014) *Paramedic Curriculum Guidance* (3rd edn). Bridgwater: College of Paramedics. Available at: https://www.collegeofparamedics.co.uk/downloads/Curriculum_Guidance_2014.pdf (accessed 18 February 2005).

Health and Care Professions Council (2014a) *Standards of Proficiency. Paramedics.* London: HCPC. Available at: http://www.hpc-uk.org/assets/documents/1000051CStandards_of_Proficiency_Paramedics.pdf (accessed 18 February 2005).

Health and Care Professions Council (2014b) *Standards of Education and Training.* London: HCPC. Available at: http://www.hcpc-uk.org.uk/aboutregistration/standards/sets/index.asp (accessed 18 January 2015).

6 LEARNING IN SIMULATION

Kevin Barrett

Simulation is somewhat of an umbrella term, as it ranges from very simple demonstration and rehearsal of clinical or interpersonal skills all the way to complex, multi-day events with other professional groups who are engaging in extremely realistic situations and settings. These may involve professional actors and be recorded.

Simulation has been a rapidly developing area in clinical education for several years and is certainly a feature of paramedic programmes in the UK; it is likely that you will meet it on the programme that you begin. The purpose of this chapter is to provide an overview of what simulation is and how it will inform your learning as a student paramedic, as well as offer you advice on how to prepare for learning by simulation.

Typically, simulation approaches involve scenarios that students have to respond to, often in teams, which are observed by the programme lecturers (the faculty) who lead the feedback and debriefing. These events are often managed in smaller groups so that the feedback and discussion are easy to manage and so that everyone has a chance to participate.

Box 6.1 What is your experience of simulation?

Student paramedic comment: There are pros and cons with simulation. You can't get volunteers to come in and have a heart attack on cue so you can practise your advanced life support skills, so the simulation manikin has to do!

The chance to practise with all the relevant kit on a dummy is good as it creates the 'procedure memory' that kicks in when you're faced with the real situation.

We also had a special house on campus which was fitted with cameras and microphones so that students could go into a 'real' home setting and face different scenarios. Each scenario was filmed so that we could all review it after and see what had been done right and what was not so right! This was a great asset and meant we got to practise lots of stuff in as close to a real way as possible.

The down side of simulation is that although it is as real as it can be, it's sometimes not real enough. When you go into a real situation you can see, hear and even smell the patient's presenting condition! We use all our senses to gain information which forms our decisions. In simulation you have to wait to be told all aspects of the patient's presentation, or you have to ask about things which in a real situation would be obvious. This can cause you to miss things or make less than good decisions at times. It's also easier to intubate a real person than a manikin – some things are simpler and easier in real life than they are when working on the plastic people.

Simulation is good for teaching you more than the 'how to' of treating patients. In simulation scenarios we discovered the dangers of becoming blinkered and focused on accomplishing some procedure or other at the expense of noticing other things going on around us which were affecting the situation. This was a really valuable lesson for when out in practice.

We had a great opportunity to go to a local fire brigade training facility where volunteers acting as patients (with gory make-up) were cut out of wrecked cars in simulated road traffic collisions. This was great in that each scenario was run in real time so you had to go with what was happening, make the right decisions about prioritising and carry out procedures whilst lots of stuff was going on around you. I was pleased that not all my patients 'died'! The real benefit was that even if you had got something wrong it was not real, but you gained knowledge of what to do differently when it is real. I grew to really like simulation scenarios and learning.

Why is simulation used in paramedic education?

Paramedic practice is quite unpredictable in nature and many learning opportunities arise infrequently and in an opportunistic manner. This is perhaps not like some other health-care professions where students can be sent to a respiratory ward, for instance, to learn about peak flow measurements or nebulisers and it is almost guaranteed that they will see these situations. To ensure that students can have exposure to seldom seen but essential elements of care delivery, simulation has a major role to play.

Paramedics use a variety of equipment to respond to urgent and emergency calls, and familiarity with all of these items is important. Simulation can demonstrate their use, as well as alternative approaches to employing them. The equipment used in manual handling manoeuvres that are required on a daily basis are a good example here. You might be given a scenario that involves access to a patient from only one side (if they are against a wall, for example) or where the space is very confined and use of the gold standard equipment is difficult, and asked to consider what steps need to be used and what other equipment might be used instead. Simulation here can reproduce real-life compromises to clinical practice, and you will always be simulating your assessment and decision-making abilities as well as use of equipment.

Safety is a huge part of the rationale for simulation. Simulation is error tolerant: mistakes or slow practice in time-pressured situations are not problematical and become good learning opportunities for yourself and colleagues. The enactments are safe for patients as no one is actually left in pain if analgesia is not considered, for example, but it is also a safe situation for you because you have the chance to learn new and sometimes complicated aspects of care delivery, knowing that no one is compromised if a mistake is made.

There is an ethical perspective that correlates to the issues of safety. We should not practise on poorly people: there is an ethical maxim called *non-maleficence* which translates as 'do no harm'. Although practice on clinical placement will always be supervised, as a student you want to be in a position where you can contribute to care in a way that is not putting a patient, yourself or staff at any risk. Alongside this, we have to acknowledge that some care interventions, such as cannulation, can be painful, and these are best first learned via simulation: students cannulate plastic arms to become accustomed to the practice.

Aside from the psycho-motor type clinical skills, some communication approaches also require a non-maleficence perspective: breaking bad news, for example. These sensitive situations can be very emotionally charged and there can be social and emotional pressures on clinicians in discussing difficult decisions and asking sensitive questions: rehearsing some of these areas via simulation can be invaluable. Indeed, receiving feedback about communication styles, including non-verbal or body language patterns, is quite a personal issue and beginning this in a structured and relatively private situation is especially helpful.

Many situations that you respond to will be surprisingly complex, and in actual clinical practice it may only be possible for the paramedic that you are working alongside to highlight a few of the areas to concentrate on to support your learning. What simulation allows is for multiple perspectives to be considered, either by repeatedly viewing discrete sections of a response through a video recording, for instance, or by having different members of the faculty deliberately look at different elements of practice. This might mean that you respond to a person who has fallen and, all at once, the way that you maintain a safe working environment, the way you approach manual handling decisions, the equipment you decide to use, the communication with the fallen person and with your team members and the thoroughness of your overall assessment of the patient are considered. This is very challenging to manage in real-time clinical practice, but simulation allows a highly structured approach to learning about potentially complex areas of care delivery and can illustrate just how multi-faceted clinical practice can be, even in everyday situations.

In some longer scenarios it is possible to address decision-making and the prioritising and re-prioritising of care delivery. These areas are highly relevant to your developing clinical practice and are quite subtle skills; simulation allows to you to comment and reflect on your own decision-making, what your rationales were and to explore alternatives with expert teachers.

One area that benefits from simulation approaches is called inter-professional learning. This encourages teams of one professional group to learn about and from another professional group. So you might undertake a set of responses with emergency department nurses to enhance the skill of concisely and accurately providing a hand-over of a patient, a skill that is being increasingly highlighted as central to good continuity of care and one that is central to paramedic practice. Additionally, you will discover from the other professionals what they need from paramedics and why.

A key term in simulation is *fidelity*, describing how realistic a situation is. An example of low fidelity is the use of simple manikins, as described in Box 6.2 by a student. They are useful in routine skills rehearsals and require little supervision or planning. 'High fidelity' usually refers to more involved situations as described in Box 6.2 by the academic and paramedic.

Box 6.2 What types of simulation experience have you been involved in?

📖 **Student paramedic response:** We did lots of simulation scenarios – anything and everything from cardiopulmonary resuscitation on manikins, to full-scale major incident scenarios with the fire brigade cutting patients out of cars.

Simulation has its drawbacks. We tend to use all of our senses when assessing our patients (apart from taste, obviously!) and a manikin doesn't always look, feel or sound like a real sick person. This sometimes gets in the way of learning. However, you can't arrange for people to come into uni and have a cardiac arrest on demand, so simulation is the best way of learning when the real thing isn't to hand.

🎓 **Academic response:** We take our students to a facility owned and run jointly by the local council, police and fire service. This is a huge area made out like a town and includes an A&E department, police station, fire station, law court, shops, restaurants, pubs, roads, houses, vehicles and even a park. We simulate incidents here for students, and feedback has been really great. Students definitely feel the benefit of being away from a classroom environment and the incidents feel more real.

🎓 **Academic response:** Many universities exploit state-of-the-art simulation to develop students' skills and leadership attributes in a safe environment, and it is essential that you engage in these activities. Macro-simulation and practical exercises allows students to explore the relationship between clinical, operational, teamwork and human factors, all of which influence service user outcome. To add realism to simulated scenarios, moulage (make-up and fake blood) is used. Simulations can be carried out at various locations to 'set the scene'; in our university we use a mock courtroom, mock ambulance, climbing wall and crime scene houses to add realism and replicate the challenges encountered in practice.

👤 **Paramedic mentor/PEd response:** Some years ago I went on a Royal College of Surgeons medicine in remote areas course. One of the exercises was a 36-hour search and rescue simulation in a wood. It was amazingly realistic, with volunteers from the casualties union taking part. The injuries looked so real you forgot that this was a simulation at all. Amazing!

One point that deserves to be highlighted in relation to paramedic practice is that the pre-hospital clinical environment needs to be simulated. It will not necessarily be the case that the skills rooms that many universities now possess (and that you will see demonstrated at open days) will be used all the time; you can expect to be in settings such as the car park, the sports field and the stairwell which present their own problem-solving challenges and are more realistic for student paramedics than the hospital ward.

Reflection: points to consider

What is actually being simulated?

- Is it the psychomotor skills and developing familiarity with equipment?
- Is it the decision-making and prioritising/re-prioritising of care?
- Is it the communication strategies needed in care delivery?
- Is it the complexities of clinical practice?

Which are the important elements that need to be high-fidelity?

- Is it the setting (e.g. an actual railway track)?
- Is it the equipment used (e.g. expensive manikins)?
- Is it that the debrief relates learning points back to actual clinical practice?

What can I expect from this way of learning?

This approach will support your learning in a number of ways. It is useful to consider your involvement with a situation in terms of being a participant (or responder) in the scenario, a patient in the scenario and as an observer of the scenario, as all present different perspectives.

- Participant: here you gain some sense of responding to the clinical scenario, familiarity with equipment and your own decision-making style. This is typically the role in which we expect most learning to occur.
- Observer: being one step removed from the practice scenario in this way allows you to become aware of peripheral issues – body

language, or how long it takes to offer analgesia for example – but can also involve you in learning how to offer feedback in some instances.

- Patient/casualty: here you have some experience of being questioned, being carried down a flight of stairs or being pulled out of a car, for example. This is invaluable because you develop sympathy for the fears that people may have simply from being in a carry chair, but also see how vital it is for patients to be kept informed of what is happening to them.

Typically, a simulation event will consist of the following stages, with some being more emphasised than others, depending on the skill set or areas of awareness that are being explored:

1   Scenario briefing. This can range from being extremely brief and vague (or even misleading, sometimes information given to paramedics responding to a 999 call is incomplete or inaccurate) to a very detailed overview of what is expected and what the intended learning outcomes are specifically trying to address.

2   Scenario enactment. This is usually either time-bound (e.g. it is stopped at 15 minutes) or outcome-bound (the response either resolves the scenario or complicates it further). The outcome-bound style of scenario is more complex but also more true to life.

3   Scenario debrief: questions. This often begins with the faculty asking the participants how they felt the scenario had run and is frequently structured to avoid any tendency towards either too much negativity or being purely congratulatory, to keep the discussion as objective as possible. Skilful faculty involvement ensures that, no matter how any individual scenario went, the learning experience is positive and participants feel supported and encouraged.

4   Scenario debrief: feedback. Normally, the faculty will have kept notes on key learning areas and a timeline of events. The timeline is extremely useful, because often our appreciation of the passage of time, particularly when we are under any form of pressure, can be inaccurate: we might think that we offered a patient oxygen almost as soon as we walked into a room, but to be told that it was after just over 5 minutes can be a revelation! This illustrates another means through which simulation can support learning; simulation can demonstrate our situational awareness. It is easy at first to be so completely engrossed in the performance of one specific element

of care that we forget other, essential aspects – for example, did anyone consider the relatives? Did anyone secure the safety of the environment?

Once a group of students are familiar with one another, there is encouragement for some of the feedback to come from those observing, too. It might be that you are given the role of studying body language or the way that medications used have been checked or disposed of, and asked to give feedback on that. This helps develop an approach for feedback to colleagues which is, of course, an unavoidable area of learning and of practice. In these instances it is understood that students have been asked to undertake the role so that the feedback is understood to be a deliberate part of the exercise and nothing personal.

& Refer to Chapters 3 and 7 for more discussion around the importance of personal reflection.

It is proposed within the literature around simulation education that about one-third of the time spent on an event is the simulation itself and that two-thirds is taken up with the debrief and discussion around the points raised during the event. These points may be the expected learning outcomes of the scenario, which are often already preset. Academics may need to facilitate discussion of alternative responses demonstrated in the scenario, which may well be unique to each enactment of a scenario, or be unique to individuals and groups.

Ideally, simulation exercises will be undertaken in small groups, perhaps under ten in a group, so that feedback can be shared in a contained setting. It can be a very supportive way of learning about all aspects of our own practice, even though it can also have a certain intensity. This intensity is managed much better in small groups and can actually help to foster a strong sense of being in a learning community, that a journey into clinical learning is being shared; it can be very motivational in this way.

Simulation events frequently see other staff (and sometimes senior students on your course) involved as part of the faculty. The advantage for your learning here is that paramedics and other clinical staff with specialist knowledge can be assembled to help deliver the exercise and ensure that feedback is as contemporaneous and as specific as possible. When senior students are involved they can address in detail the issues as they may affect the student perspective.

How can I make the most of opportunities to learn in simulation?

When you know that there will be a simulation day or scenario as part of your programme you can maximise what you take from the approach:

- Be an active learner. If you are given the scenarios beforehand, study them and clarify areas that you are unsure about. If an illness is going to be encountered, read in advance around that, or if there is equipment to be used that you are unfamiliar with try and review it prior to the day.
- During the day, take notes. A lot can happen in one scenario and you may well want to ask questions of the faculty. Afterwards, to guide your own learning, you will want to follow up with reading around points raised that were either interesting or unclear for you on the day; at university students are expected to be able to guide their own learning. With these points in mind, bring paper and pen or tablet to make your notes on!
- Volunteer! There is always some trepidation at first, but everyone benefits from the lessons to be learned, and well-managed simulations acknowledge that the learning is shared.

> **Box 6.3 What advice would you give students to make the most of this way of learning?**
>
> 📖 **Student paramedic response:** Repetition cements learning: keep practising on manikins and going to scenario days. Just as doing a certain sport creates what athletes call 'muscle memory', so simulation practice creates procedure memory.
>
> 🔔 **Paramedic response:** Working in health care, simulation is something you get used to. I have taken part in a large-scale road traffic collisions and major incident simulation. This was incredibly useful as it is, thankfully, not something routinely seen. It gave me a chance to see how I would feel initially managing such a situation, therefore preparing me for this kind of event. Initially, I always feel a bit self-conscious when taking part in a scenario. In my experience assessors try to make them seem as realistic as possible and you soon forget people are watching. Assessment through scenarios continues once you are registered. Most ambulance trusts have an advanced life

support scenario as part of their interview process. Further scenarios are used for professional updates throughout your working life.

Academic response: As good as simulation can be, it is not without its limitations. In reality, we can often glean enough information about our patients to conduct a primary survey from the door and make the decision whether or not the patient is time-critical. In simulation this is often not the case. Make sure you ask, ask, ask! If the assessor does not proffer enough information, ask about what you are seeing, feeling and hearing. Get into the habit of verbalising everything. This can be initially very challenging as it feels unnatural and does not happen in practice, but it is an invaluable skill to learn. It will show the assessor your thought processes and give a good indication of why you are treating a patient in a certain way. I liken it to sitting a maths test – it is not enough to write down the correct answer; you need to show your working out. Even if the simulation is not as real as you would like it to be, remember it is an excellent way of learning a systematic approach to patient assessment and treatment.

CASE STUDY 6.1

Final-year paramedic and midwifery students were grouped together into a number of teams and had to respond to a number of homebirth situations. The students had to rely on each other's skill set, the different equipment they have available and to make decisions as a team about moving the pregnant woman onto an ambulance.

The debrief for each team exposed similar issues: that communication was paramount and being clear about who needed to take the lead during separate stages of the scenario mattered to both professional groups and to the safety of mother and child. This sharing or alternating of the clinical lead role is an advanced and refined area, and simulation allowed some confidence to be developed about strategies that would clarify who ought to be directing care and considering the next step.

Student paramedics were able to develop some confidence that they need not be embarrassed about assessing the woman in labour, something that normal social conventions would dictate against, but student midwives were able to be quite clear about the importance of knowing how far the baby's head had appeared and what this meant in terms of imminent delivery. This type of communication across and between disciplines is invaluable and can be accessed through simulated scenarios.

In summary, simulation approaches are, in fact, unavoidable in clinical education. They occur all the time in all manner of guises, from moving and handling demonstrations to physical assessment exams. Whether simulation involves low- or high-tech approaches, what matters most is your own engagement.

Suggested reading/websites

Riley, R.H. (2010) *Manual of Simulation in Healthcare*. Oxford: Oxford University Press.

The Association for Simulated Practice in Healthcare has a useful website at http://www.aspih.org.uk/. ASPiH is a not-for-profit company limited by guarantee. It is a membership association formed through the merger of the National Association of Medical Simulators and the Clinical Skills Network. It aims to enable a wider sharing of knowledge, expertise, and educational innovation related to simulated practice across the health-care professions.

7 HOW CAN I LINK MY ACADEMIC STUDIES AND CLINICAL PRACTICE?

Several points have already been made about the use of reflection, independent study and guided study. All of these recognised approaches should help you make the link between theory and practice.

⋋ Refer to Chapter 3 for discussion about the use of reflective practice and Chapter 5 for detailed ideas for making the most of your independent and guided study time.

> **Reflection: points to consider**
>
> Think of a time when your studies have directly helped you in everyday life.
>
> What worked well?
>
> Could you have made more of the learning experience?

It may also be useful to read specific books on study skills and reflection. It is important that you find texts that suit your reading style and that you find informative and interesting; a selection of reading material is provided in the suggested reading at the end of this chapter.

Handy hints to help you link theory and practice

You are reading this text to learn more about being a student paramedic, so it makes sense for you to read ideas directly from students on this matter, with opinions and additional suggestions from academics and paramedics/PEds.

The comments in Box 7.1 describe a number of different approaches and may give you some ideas and help you understand the importance of making the links between theory and practice.

Box 7.1 What strategies would you suggest to successfully link your academic studies and clinical practice? What worked for you?

📖 **Student paramedic response:** I took a couple of relevant books on shift with me so that after each job we attended I could look up things like the causes, complications, treatment of the patient's condition and learn more. Seeing a patient with a condition you've read about cements understanding, and reading up on things you've seen on placement develops knowledge and decision-making.

I would also keep a note of each job we went to so that I could look up relevant aspects of it later when I could search the literature on it and gain more insight. Obviously you're talking with your mentor about each job, getting their reasoning and understanding of it. I found also that my mentors would ask me lots of things about current thinking on treatments, etc. as they knew we were getting the most up-to-date thinking on it in our lectures and they wanted to learn from me as much as I was learning from them. This was a really good aspect of my placement experience. It wasn't just a case of the student sitting at the feet of the master – we shared the learning experience.

🚨 **Paramedic mentor/PEd response:** Students often ask why they need to study some subjects in such depth, anatomy, physiology and pathophysiology being the most common. 'Why do we need to know this?' is a common question. When students are on placement and are exposed to a particular medical condition for the first time, they already have a good understanding of exactly what is happening and why. It is at this point that many students have said how glad they were they had the underpinning knowledge to understand what was going on.

🚨 **Paramedic mentor/PEd response:** My mentor reviewed patients' conditions with me afterwards and quizzed me on anatomy, physiology, altered physiology, treatment options and medications. This was never done in a negative way. Often we used to work things out together or she used to teach me certain aspects. As a student, I disliked this approach, mainly because I was self-conscious and really did not want to get anything wrong. How crazy – I was learning a new job, of course I would get things wrong or not know something. But I realise now how this approach really made me go away and learn the things I could not answer and did not know. It is a similar approach that I use with my students now. I also try to widen the scope of subjects to areas such as sociology and psychology, as many of our calls are to people with social or psychological issues. It is not just physical illness that this job is about; as paramedic mentors we need to make sure we assess our students on the holistic range of problems that patients have. Each call usually has an element of physical, social and psychological issues that can be explored and linked to theory.

🎓 **Academic response:** It is a fact that students will engage more with subjects they feel have relevance to practice. As a lecturer I take every opportunity to point out how the academic subjects are relevant to practice and try to give good examples. Don't be afraid to ask your lecturers to point out the relevance of subjects – you may be surprised how even the subjects that are perceived as the driest academic ones have hidden relevance.

Using jobs you have attended as starting points for your own study and further research is also a very good way to link academic studies to practice. When one actually sees a medical condition much of the underpinning knowledge will click into place.

It is good to think more widely about sources of expertise and information. Our patients are a major source of information, and they may know their condition in more detail than we do, especially if it is something quite unique and rare. This is explained well by Case Study 7.1.

CASE STUDY 7.1

I remember attending a job involving a little girl who had fallen from height. On checking her pupils I found them to be grossly bilaterally dilated. This just didn't make sense as the rest of her signs and symptoms did not add up. It was only when mum arrived and she informed me the little girl had a condition called 'aniridia' (the absence of an iris) that this made sense. It was interesting for me to be able to research this condition when I got home and is a good example of how theory can directly link to practice.

As Case Study 7.1 clearly shows, practice and theory are inextricably linked. No matter how long you have been a registered paramedic, there will be things you come across that require you to *hit the books* and remind yourself of something or learn about something new. So never be afraid of learning from your patient; it is not a sign of weakness or lack of competence. If your programme involves block placements, it is wise to try and keep in touch with academic staff at your institution while on placement. This may take the form of occasional e-mails or more formal one-to-one meetings to discuss your general progress or any specific issue that is of concern to you at the time.

Textbooks will often list signs and symptoms of certain conditions, but it is wise to remember that patients will not present in such a textbook fashion. Symptoms and signs may vary, and your role is often one of a detective, trying to piece together clues that you collect from the patients, significant others and physical data. Often you may need to refer to textbooks to help explain the variation from the normal symptoms/signs that you would have expected, or the interaction of different disease processes. This will add to your expertise and may help you in the future, with other patients presenting with similar signs and symptoms.

This aim of this chapter was to provide you with some ideas about how others have approached linking clinical practice with theory. Do not be averse to trying other strategies. Speak to your colleagues and mentor/PEds – they may have some innovative ideas that you can try for yourself. Linking the two together generally also strengthens your ability to study independently and gives you the ability to visualise your patient and not just see a signs and symptoms table in a textbook. This generally makes it easier to learn and is more interesting for many students.

Suggested reading

Bolton, G.E.J. (2014) *Reflective Practice. Writing and Professional Development* (4th edn). London: Sage.

Richardson, M. (2012) Reflective practice in relation to pre-hospital care. In A.Y. Blaber (ed.) *Foundations for Paramedic Practice: A Theoretical Perspective* (2nd edn). Maidenhead: Open University Press.

Rolfe, G., Jasper, M. and Freshwater, D. (2010) *Critical Reflection in Practice: Generating Knowledge for Care* (2nd edn). Basingstoke: Palgrave Macmillan.

Sibson, L. (2009) An introduction to reflective practice. *Journal of Paramedic Practice*, 1(3): 121–125.

Willis, S. (2010) Becoming a reflective practitioner: frameworks for pre-hospital professionals. *Journal of Paramedic Practice*, 2(5): 212–216.

PART 3
Placement: preparing for and making the most of it

Part 2 of this book has been primarily focused upon your academic studies, but this is inextricably linked to your experiences and learning in clinical practice as a student paramedic. You cannot consider one without the other; consequently there have been some brief suggestions made about the practice environment. However, Part 3 is predominantly related to your experience in the practice environment.

PART 3
Placement: preparing for and making the most of it

8 IS PRACTICE WHAT YOU THINK IT IS GOING TO BE?

Reflection: points to consider

Before you read this chapter, make a list of the key words you associate with *student paramedic practice experience*.

You will probably be most looking forward to what is commonly called *going out to practice*. Many students find this the most exciting prospect of being a student paramedic. For some the reality is vastly different than they expected, while others feel very prepared and it is exactly as they envisaged it would be, as highlighted by the diversity of comments made by students in Chapter 1. One thing that is certain is that no one can predict what you are going to see or experience during shifts in any clinical environment, the ambulance service being no exception. Your safety and that of your colleagues is of utmost importance and you will be provided with safety guidance information. Case Study 8.1 has been included to help dispel the myth that all ambulance service work is action-packed and to highlight the importance of communication.

CASE STUDY 8.1

I remember having to tell a 90-year-old lady that we had not been successful at resuscitating her husband. I had been talking to her while the resuscitation attempt was in progress in the room next door. Among so many other things, I knew they had been married for 66 years, knew about their family and how they had met. I found this one of the hardest things to do, yet one of the most rewarding. I had been sitting talking, comforting, explaining, discussing all manner of subjects for over an hour. I had connected with the lady, as I had the time to get to know her. I found it extremely difficult to leave her when it was time for us to go.

For many of the 'non-initiated' the job of a paramedic is all about blue lights and road traffic collisions. This is *not* the case. A huge part of the job is being able to provide comfort and reassurance to vulnerable (often elderly and lonely) people. Some of my most satisfying jobs have been clinically insignificant but I have gone away knowing I made a huge difference to that person at that time.

The emotions explained in Case Study 8.1 help to explain the diversity of the role and highlight that while the call was an emergency, the role of each professional attending may be extremely diverse and require very different approaches to the situation.

It may be that not all of your clinical experience will be on a frontline 999 vehicle with blue flashing lights. There is much more to the ambulance service, and answering 999 calls is just one aspect of the service that any ambulance trust provides. Indeed, depending on your programme, you may also spend a significant amount of time in non-ambulance service clinical areas, observing the role of paramedics and other clinical staff working in these areas.

Types of ambulance service placement

Clinical/placement areas that encompass primary, acute, urgent, community and emergency care environments provide the opportunity for learning outcomes to be achieved and can be considered as relevant to the student paramedic experience. This section of the chapter will outline the types of ambulance placements considered relevant by the College of Paramedics (2014). You must remember that it is not possible to visit/work in all of the placements listed in this chapter during your time as a student paramedic. The opportunities will vary from university to university and between programmes of study.

Student paramedic comment: On our programme each student was allocated ambulance placements at two different base stations, one urban and one more rural, which gave us experience of all types of patients/environments. I thought the rural one would be quiet and uneventful compared to the urban station, but often the quaint town on a Sunday afternoon was busier than the city on a Friday night! I even went to an armed siege, complete with riot squad! It just goes to show you never know what could happen on a shift – that's one of the things I love about the job.

We went to a lot of patients with mental health issues. I found that these patients were the ones I felt the most empathy for, as although we could help them with an immediate problem we felt fairly powerless to make a lasting, long-term difference for them. I'd say we go to more patients with social or mental health issues than patients with trauma. Being a paramedic is not all about running from car crashes to cardiac arrests all day; it's about going to people who often didn't know who else to call – which doesn't mean it's not important or rewarding. You just need to like people and have loads of patience, empathy and a willingness to do the best you can for them.

As Case Study 8.1 and the above student paramedic comment illustrate, the patients you will care for may be experiencing a different kind of crisis than you might have envisaged the ambulance service would be called upon to manage and help with. It is therefore important that programmes address all aspects of care, and not just focus on physical aspects. To help programme teams achieve this, other professionals with expertise, such as mental health nurses, may be asked for input into your programme. This is something that your mentors/PEds undertaking in-house ambulance service training courses may not have had the benefit of, so make the most of the expertise around you and learn as much as possible.

The ambulance service offers a wide variety of experiences, some of which you may find a surprise. Table 8.1 details the types of ambulance service placements that the College of Paramedics (2014) recommends as being suitable for student paramedics. Often a programme structure is such that at certain points in the programme it may be more appropriate to undertake certain types of placements. For example, it may be more beneficial for a student paramedic who is undertaking or has just completed their physical assessment module/unit to work with a solo responder so they can gain more experience and use their physical assessment skills more consistently. Or it may be that your PEd/mentor is a solo

Table 8.1 Types of ambulance service placements that may be included in paramedic programmes (College of Paramedics 2014)

Ambulance emergency unit – a blue-light ambulance or 999 vehicle
Single response vehicles
Specialist operation units
Emergency operation control centres (999 and 111 systems)
Non-emergency services

responder, so you naturally will spend more time on this type of vehicle than your colleagues, but it is also important you spend a large part of your time on an emergency frontline (999) vehicle.

It is worth experiencing the role and pressure of the emergency operation control centre early in your studies and then revisiting it once you have a more comprehensive appreciation of your role. Again, appreciating other people's roles is important to understand their pressures, priorities and working environment. Assessing and taking information without seeing who you are talking to is very different, and requires different communication skills than meeting a person face to face. It is very easy to criticise each other, but an appreciation of the difficulties of communication and an understanding of roles are vital for a cohesive and efficient service for patients.

Specialist operation units, referred to in Table 8.1, are included so that students can appreciate the role and use of paramedics as part of these services. These may include British Association for Immediate Care Schemes (BASICS), hazardous area response teams, urban search and rescue, baby/neonate emergency transfer units, and helicopter medical services. It is highly probable that students will not be able to secure placements with these specialist teams, but you may have visits or lectures from people from these teams as part of your programme. As you can imagine, these services are small and make up a small part of any ambulance service, so rotating large numbers of student paramedics through them is usually impossible.

The role of non-emergency services in Table 8.1 refers to the role and operation of patient transport services' delivery of care and transportation

(College of Paramedics 2014: 45). This may involve admissions to or discharges from hospital and observation/implementation of moving and handling skills. Again communication skills are an invaluable part of this learning opportunity, should you have the chance to undertake a placement in your local patient transport service, if it is not run by a private company.

Whatever placement experience you have in the ambulance service, at some point you will be required to undertake various shift patterns.

Shift work

This was briefly mentioned in Chapter 3, but requires more attention, as it can be the difference between students enjoying their role and finding it too much and giving up their studies. Inevitably student paramedics will encounter shift work at some point in their careers. The vast majority of programmes involve students working shifts from early on, usually year 1. Some may not involve that much shift work. Whatever your programme does in respect of shift work, it is certain that your first employed role as a paramedic in an ambulance service will expect you to undertake the variety of shift patterns designated by your trust, as the responses in Box 8.1 explain.

> **Box 8.1 In your experience, what shifts are allocated to students? Does this change when you are registered?**
>
> **Paramedic response:** During my time as a student I had an easy-going mentor that I could text and arrange shifts with. For a placement I needed to give my availability a month or so in advance, and they were still flexible around my part-time job, etc. Since registration, and, more importantly, employment, there is little choice. My current rota has me working three out of four weekends and I'm lucky if I do less than 50% nights in a month. Unfortunately, the unsocial shifts are where the demand is and if you choose to work for a trust where you know you will be relief staff, read your contract thoroughly and understand these implications, it's quite a shock to the system!
>
> **Paramedic mentor/PEd response:** In most cases students will 'mirror' the shift pattern of their on-road mentor. This is usually a full

range of shifts following a rota. This can change when a newly qualified paramedic is employed by a trust as in some cases the new
staff member will start on a relief line. This can be challenging as the
shifts do not follow a pattern and shorter notice is given as to what
hours will be required. This said, relief positions are usually only
temporary until a permanent line becomes available and are a good
way of 'getting a foot in the door'.

Paramedic mentor/PEd response: A full range of shift work is
required throughout the programme of study, and you shouldn't wait
until you qualify to do your first night shift or your first weekend or
bank holiday. Having said this, take your time to adjust to odd shift
times and don't rush into working continuous nights or having quick
turnarounds, swapping from days to nights or vice versa. It will take
a bit of getting used to, but take it slowly and by the time you qualify
you will be set to go. Your shift pattern when registered will be different and may be more intense, but your previous experience of the
range of shifts will make the transition much easier.

Box 8.1 highlights the various approaches to shift work that the student
paramedic may encounter. The responses also help to explain the variety
of shift patterns that you may be expected to work and how this may help
to prepare you for employment. The difficulty of shift work should not be
underestimated, and the following comments help to explain how important it is to develop your own strategy for coping with shift work.

Student paramedic comment: Shift work is difficult, especially the
switch between night and day shifts. I still haven't got used to these –
apparently it takes about ten years! It can take a couple of days to
reset your body clock after night shifts. Different people have different methods for dealing with it. Some stay up for the whole day after
a night shift, others get a couple of hours then make themselves get
up – you will find what works for you, but you can feel pretty jetlagged
for a while until you find your way of dealing with it.

Paramedic comment: One year into my career I'm fairly used to
nights. I have a pattern which I generally follow. Before my first night
I try to lie in as long as possible, usually about 10:30, then go about

my day as normal, including some form of exercise. Arrive at work about 20 minutes early to ensure there is time for a coffee. I can then sleep solidly between the rest of my nights. If I finish on time, I may even get up an hour earlier, for a jog after a few nights. I struggle more with day shifts, I've never been a morning person! Again, coffee is my answer; I always have a Thermos and a couple of sachets of cappuccino in my bag.

Academic comment: I would disagree with the comment above saying getting used to shifts takes about ten years. I had no problem with early (07.00–14.30) or late shifts (14.00–22.00) or 12-hour shifts (08.00–20.00). However, I never got used to night shifts. We used to be allocated seven nights at a time. I just used to manage them as best I could, and that wasn't very well. I used to dread the rota including them, write off that week of my life and the one following it, as it used to take me three or four days to get back into a regular sleep pattern. Some of my colleagues only worked night shifts, and declined to work day shifts, if they had the choice.

There is no one-size-fits-all advice that can be given about managing or coping with shift patterns. The comments from all contributors point to the fact that you need to try it for yourself, as the responses in Box 8.2 help to explain.

Box 8.2 What are the difficulties and/or pleasures of shift work?

🚨 **PEd response:** I used to love working night shifts. The world is a totally different place at night, and some of my most interesting and challenging jobs seemed to occur on nights. There also seemed to be more camaraderie between staff on night shifts. Last, but not least, going home to a warm bed on a cold and rainy Monday morning when everyone else had to be up for work was one of my small but significant pleasures!

🚨 **Paramedic response:** There are many pros and cons to shift work. Many people in the ambulance service say they aren't built for 9–5, and this is true for me. The biggest difficulty I have working shifts is missing out on social events, particularly at weekends. You can guarantee if you make plans after work, you'll be so late off it won't be worth attending. I have had a few occasions where this has happened and I've found myself really upset at missing family members' birthdays, etc. Now I've learnt my lesson, I rarely arrange to do anything after work; if I do, I warn people involved that I may not actually make it or may get there late. Things that I don't want to miss, I book off with annual leave.

My favourite thing about shifts is having so much time off. Working a 12-hour day is long, but you do three or four and then the week is yours. I get so much done on my days off, time to myself and to enjoy my hobbies.

The wide variation in personal opinion regarding shift work should be appreciated by the reader having read the variation in comments and responses included in this chapter. Shift work, particularly at night, is a bit like Marmite, you either love it or hate it! You need to make up your own mind.

Reflection: point to consider

Write down your own list of pros and cons of working unsocial hours.

It is likely that you will have the opportunity to also experience non-ambulance placements whilst studying as well as ambulance placements.

Non-ambulance service placements

There are guidelines for suitable student paramedic placements, provided by the College of Paramedics (2014) for HEIs and NHS ambulance trusts. The list is extensive, as can be seen in Table 8.2, and the College of Paramedics (2014) also explains the potential value of the learning experience from these clinical areas. The availability of these areas to student paramedics may depend on a variety of political and local factors and (most crucially) the number of other health-care students already placed in these areas, as part of their programme of study.

Table 8.2 Types of non-ambulance service placements that may be included in paramedic programmes (College of Paramedics 2014)

Operating theatres/day procedure unit	Emergency department
Obstetric/midwifery unit	Cardiac care/cardiac catheterisation unit (CCU)
Minor injuries/illness unit	Intensive care unit (ICU) or high-dependency unit
Medical assessment unit	Mental health unit/community mental health team
Paediatric department/ward	Out-of-hours unscheduled care
Surgical assessment unit	Allied health teams (physiotherapists, occupational therapists, community health teams)
Other emergency services, e.g. police, traffic police, fire service, coastguard, RAF Search and Rescue, Royal National Lifeboat Institute	

Occasionally, other health-care students (nurses, midwives) will have the opportunity to work on ambulances, but predominantly these opportunities are afforded to student paramedics. The same applies to student midwives, for example, who need the majority of their practice hours to be spent in midwifery-focused clinical areas. It may be, therefore, that there is not the capacity to accept student paramedics in other clinical areas within your locality. It is very much a situation that varies from year to year, depending on local demand. Your programme teams will work closely with university placement teams and try their best to secure alternative placements where possible.

Non-ambulance placements can help the student to gain an element of insight and witness other health professionals working with varying patient groups. Placements in non-ambulance areas serve to enhance relationships, teamwork and communication across professions and within the workplace. Students must experience inter-professional working to develop the required competencies essential to work within a collaborative workforce.

Table 8.2 lists appropriate non-ambulance service placement opportunities for the student paramedic. It will not be the case that all students will experience all of the placements listed in Table 8.2. As mentioned above, there will be local variation and, in some cases, limited availability of such placements.

Many of the areas mentioned in Table 8.2 are an opportunity to improve your communication skills with patients, as in some of the areas the patients you will encounter will not be seriously ill and you will have the opportunity to take your time, assess them and talk to them. This would not be appropriate in areas such as a CCU or ICU, but instead there you will see the work that goes on once the ambulance crew has handed over the patient and have the opportunity to extend your knowledge in relation to the specifics of the patient's condition.

There are a wide variety of learning opportunities available by exploring the wider NHS and the roles of other health professionals. The more you develop your knowledge of the NHS as a whole and the services available in your locality, the more you can pass this information on to your patients and help them to potentially make informed choices regarding their health in the future. Your understanding of what happens in these areas may help to alleviate your patients' anxiety at a point in the future, so these placements are equally as valuable as ambulance service opportunities. Box 8.3 includes responses relating to the benefits of non-ambulance service placements.

Box 8.3 What are the benefits of undertaking non-ambulance service focused placements?

📖 **Student paramedic response:** CCU was great, I got to see how the doctors treat cardiac patients from the point paramedics bring them in, to the point the patient leaves hospital. This was really useful as it gives you insight into the care a patient will get once you've handed them over and you can use this knowledge to reassure relatives and friends of future patients.

Maternity was my favourite placement, mainly because the staff were so nice and really enthusiastic towards paramedics getting involved. I got to help deliver 12 babies (including at a Caesarean section) – really rewarding stuff. Lots of paramedics seem scared of maternity jobs, but this placement gave me a confidence that I will be able to handle these jobs well, as and when they come.

I found that if you put yourself out as a student when on placement in hospitals, offering to help make beds or hand out the patients' dinners (even clean the bed pans) then the staff take notice and really appreciate you being there, which then makes them want to give you their time and create opportunities for you to learn more. Some students didn't do much to help if it didn't include what they were there to do; as a result they didn't get to see much. You get out of placement what you're willing to put in.

🎓 **Academic response:** Non-ambulance based placements are incredibly valuable not just in clinical terms, but in allowing us to understand what a patient experiences after they leave our care. When we 'deliver' a patient to the ED it is the end of our journey, but the start of theirs (often a very long one). It also gives us an appreciation of the roles of other health professionals and makes for good working relationships in the future.

Attending any placement can be a stressful experience, so it is important that you feel prepared. Ensure that you are clear about both your responsibilities and those of the registered clinician, in respect of the placement environment and any assessment processes. The following section of the chapter provides some useful suggestions to help reduce the pressure and stress you may feel prior to attending non-ambulance service placements.

Preparing for non-ambulance service placements

Any change you experience can be a difficult time. Most non-ambulance placements will occur after year 1 of your programme, by which time you will be comfortable when in ambulance placements. Going to a different clinical or community area will be strange and a different experience. Your time in these areas may be limited, ranging from a few days to a few weeks; they are unlikely to be any longer. It is therefore important that you are ready to go to the area, have an idea what to expect and start getting involved quickly, otherwise it will be over before you know it.

Reflection: points to consider

Make a list of things you want to see, experience and learn about while you are in your non-ambulance placement. This will depend on the type of area, so think carefully.

Talk to other students who have already been to these areas, and focus on what learning opportunities there are.

Go to the placement with a clear idea of what you want to learn while you are there. This will help to demonstrate your enthusiasm when you first arrive.

In order to help you prepare, ask your lecturers and/or placement team for any books and local information provided by the placement. Some placement areas provide information and workbooks for other health-care students to look at before they start the placement: would this be useful? Talk to your lecturers about what they think you should learn or focus on while in the placement; they may be able to direct you to guided study they have prepared. Some programmes may provide you with clear learning outcomes. The following comments and Case Study 8.2 help to explain the difficulties of attending non-ambulance placements, but also the immense benefits of working with a multi-professional team.

Student paramedic comment: As well as ambulance placements we had placements in hospitals. We did a week in a cardiac care unit (CCU), two weeks in theatres and two weeks in maternity. Each placement was different. It's difficult to prepare for these placements other than by reading up on the skills you are hoping to practise and develop. You can get a varied response from the staff there, ranging from those really keen to help you to those who might see you as someone getting in the way. Consequently, it can take a couple of days to find your feet on some placements. I struggled with the theatre placement because of this. Everyone was busy getting on with their work and left me to find my own way around, but in the end I met some paramedic-friendly anaesthetists who took me under their wing and taught me loads. I discovered the notice board where they put up the theatre lists detailing which operations were being carried out each day, and worked out a plan of where to be, at what time, to step in and ask to help with cannulating and intubating. I had to be proactive and push myself forward, but it paid off as I developed these skills and also got to observe during some amazing operations. Seeing 'living' anatomy opened up before you is totally different from a textbook diagram or photo of an anatomical specimen.

Academic comment: I had heard many horror stories of how unfriendly theatre staff could be to paramedics on placement. I was determined to make the best of my placement so arrived on my first day in theatre with some large tins of biscuits and a big smile. I pushed myself forward and was friendly to everyone. The result was that I had a great time and was allowed exposure to a whole range of extra experiences such as being allowed to assist on paediatric lists and stay to observe operations.

It is difficult to settle in quickly, but a positive, enthusiastic attitude will be noticed by staff and may be the difference between a rewarding and informative experience and one that is lacking in learning opportunities. As Case Study 8.2 clearly explains, even a short two-week placement can have an impact on your own individual practice, teamwork and help to improve your patient care.

CASE STUDY 8.2

I attended an ED for two weeks as part of my student paramedic placement system. I had predetermined thoughts and ideas of what I wanted to achieve from this placement and preconceptions on how I thought an ED would function in comparison to pre-hospital care and being in the back of an ambulance.

The biggest thing I learnt from this placement was that although we step in and out of an ED environment on a daily basis with patients and communicate with staff, the lack of awareness and understanding of roles from both sides is huge. I had the opportunity to speak with different staff members to gain an insight into what we all do. We all think that the care we are providing patients in our environment is correct, which it is, but it massively increased my understanding of little things we can do pre-hospitally that will help make the transition of care easier for ED staff and the patient. For example, if we are with a patient who will potentially require cardiac intervention, cannulating a patient on the left-hand side when possible will allow a doctor easier access to perform his intervention as he/she will need to be on the right side of the patient. If we are going to immobilise a patient, removing things from pockets and belts will mean the patient can go for X-rays and scans more quickly and without delay. Additionally, when we write our paperwork, we may use a range of abbreviations that in our environment we all understand, but other people reading our paperwork may not use the same ones, so keeping our language simple stops any confusion.

I also learnt just how busy EDs are, and quite simply staff in these environments deal with a hundred things at once. We see one patient at a time, but staff in ED are responsible for the care of a number of patients at any one time. It was also interesting to learn the avail-ability of resources a hospital has – by that I mean that there are specialists available for most circumstances – and how limited we are in the community.

During this placement I gained massive exposure to and experience of patient care and developed confidence in my ability to gain a patient history, as this is done repeatedly with every patient. My record-keeping abilities developed, along with my communication skills. Communication varies from when we see patients experiencing their emergency to how they communicate once in a hospital environ-ment, and this was interesting to witness. Finally, my confidence grew in skills, such as taking bloods and cannulating. We attempt these skills in challenging environments under extreme pressure, as the main focus is to deliver emergency and life-saving drugs, but in a hospital you are able to develop these skills in a more relaxed and controlled environment.

It is important to notice how the contributor in Case Study 8.2 has appre-ciated the wider role of the ED. Small points about practice have been mentioned too, such as removing keys from pockets, and how this simple act can have an impact on the patient's journey. As the contributor wisely states, understanding and appreciating each other's roles is potentially one of the most valuable lessons that can be learnt from non-ambulance service placements.

Reflection: points to consider

At the beginning of this chapter you were asked to write a list of words you associated with student paramedic practice experience. Go back to your list of words and think about them again, in light of what you have read.

Were your expectations accurate in the areas that have been discussed in this chapter?

This chapter has discussed some idiosyncrasies of student paramedic ambulance and non-ambulance service placements, and what you can expect if you are lucky enough to have non-ambulance placements included in your programme. The next chapter will consider the care of the patient and the interaction you, as a student paramedic, may have with patients and their families.

Suggested reading

College of Paramedics (2014) *Paramedic Curriculum Guidance* (3rd edn). Bridgwater: College of Paramedics. Available at: https://www. collegeofparamedics.co.uk/downloads/Curriculum_Guidance_2014.pdf (accessed 18 February 2005).

Review your programme reading lists, guides, workbooks, and information that may be available pertaining to your placement.

9 WHAT YOU WANTED TO DO THIS FOR – THE CARE OF PATIENTS AND THEIR FAMILIES

In this chapter we will consider the contact you have with patients and the way you care for them, and also the ways that the six Cs, put together by the NHS, should shape how we care.

You will have direct contact with patients and their significant others from quite early on in your programme of study. You will not be responsible for carrying out hands-on care initially, but your mentor/PEd may wish to move you out of the role of observer to be involved in some aspect of care quite early on in your clinical experience. This period of time will be different for each student, but do expect it. The role of student paramedic is not a passive one, of observation only. It is challenging, dynamic and one that involves you in the patient's care and that of their family from fairly early on.

Your mentor/PEd will be the person who directs your learning in the clinical environment, when you are in the presence of patients and families. The mentor/PEd, usually in negotiation with you, decides what you can and cannot do. How this is decided is explained by some mentors/ PEds in Box 9.1.

Box 9.1 How do you decide how much patient responsibility to give a student paramedic?

Mentor response: I would try to work a few shifts with my student, ask them questions, so I can assess their knowledge base. I would also ask if they had any care experience. This is not always a positive, as students can bring with them bad habits and incorrect information. So I may need to spend time with my student unlearning incorrect, inappropriate practice. I will start with establishing if my student can start a conversation with a patient who is not time-critical. For the first few months it may be that I can get on with doing things, like the observations, while my student starts conversations and gathers personal information. I will support the student but reverse the roles, as usually the student will choose to take the role that they are most comfortable with; they need to develop confidence and competence in all aspects of the paramedic role. Over time, this builds to a senior student running the job, with me supervising them, in the background, and butting in when the student needs it or the patient's condition requires it.

PEd response: I initially found it very difficult to relinquish *control* to my student. At that time, this was due to my inexperience as a mentor. As time went on and I became an experienced mentor, I found this became easier. Particularly in the second year of placement, I would adopt a more supportive role to my student, acting, where appropriate, as an assistant and allowing them to take the lead. Deciding how much responsibility to allow a student obviously also depends on the individual and the quality of his/her progress. I was very lucky throughout my career as a mentor to have students who responded to my approach and made fantastic progress. I always let my students know I would never let them flounder or put them in a position where they could do anything wrong. By making this clear from the start the students felt much more confident to try taking the lead.

Mentors/PEds may have varying approaches to mentoring and consider different aspects when allocating students responsibility. What is important is that you do not attempt to do anything that you have not previously been shown how to do in university or that you are still not comfortable doing.

Important point

Student paramedics will always be closely supervised.

The setting of your placements will vary. The role of community health-care professionals is different from that of hospital-based staff; you are responsible for entering people's homes on a regular basis.

Reflection: points to consider

What do you think are the main points to consider when you enter a patient's home?

Would you act any differently if attending a patient in the local shop?

Entering a person's home

Many of your encounters with patients will take place in their own homes. The first thing to remember is that you are being invited into their home and as such are a guest. You do not have a right to be there. If at any point the patient or family ask you to leave you are legally obliged to do so.

Student comment: I've met a range of responses when entering a patient's home. Sometimes the door is opened by a person who appears really calm and unconcerned to see you, and you then find out they are the patient! At other times people are obviously worried and usher you straight in to where the patient is waiting. You know it's a potentially serious job when a relative or friend runs out to meet you whilst you're still parking the ambulance.

Often people call an ambulance when they are really distressed. Calming and reassuring relatives as well as the patient is often one of the first things needed. Sometimes relatives are angry or a bit shouty; usually this is because they are scared themselves and don't know what to do. They have to release their emotion somehow and at times it can be aimed at you. Staying polite but firm presents confidence and often calms the situation. The same relatives are then normally really apologetic about their response to you once they see everything is under control. Having said that, it's quite rare that a relative will start telling you what they think you should do. Most people instantly see you as *in charge* of the situation once you've arrived. I guess a lot of their distress is to do with not knowing what they should be doing for their relative, so once you arrive it's a relief to them that they don't have to manage the situation any more.

The various examples given by the student in the above comments highlight some of the responses you may encounter when going into a patient's home. The one tool that may be the difference between defusing a difficult aggressive encounter and making the situation worse is talking and, more widely, communication strategies.

Talking to your patient

This is where your previous life experience of talking to a variety of different people will serve you well. The value of verbal and non-verbal communication skills cannot be overestimated. Ultimately, your professional role is calmly and in a non-authoritarian way to take control of the situation, assess both the situation and your patient, administer the correct treatment and manage the patient's condition and situation. While doing all of this you need to try to reduce anxiety, tension and instil confidence in all who are present. A tall order, but remember you have a period of time in which to reach this point. It will not happen overnight and no one will expect you to be good at all aspects immediately. Box 9.2 provides some suggestions that you may find useful.

Box 9.2 Some tips about how to start a conversation with a patient and/or family member

🎓 **Academic response:** Use the cues around you – things like photographs can be a great starting point to help distract your patient and take their mind off their illness/injury, providing they are not critically ill. It may also help you start a conversation. Make sure that this is appropriate, though; in an emergency situation or when the patient is very ill this may not be the best approach. Your first priority is to gather information and data about their physical condition. Make sure you take your lead from your mentor/PEd.

📖 **Student paramedic response:** I always introduce myself and ask the patient's name (apart from easing tension, if the patient can speak to you it shows their airway is probably clear).

Communication skills and a professional manner are probably the most important things you need. How you say something is as important as what you say. Being able to talk calmly when others in the room are losing it; being authoritative but polite when you need to be; being able to effectively coach a patient who is having a panic attack, etc. – it's all about having a calm professional manner and giving the appearance that you have everything under control, even if inside you're wondering what the hell to do next!

Paramedic/PEd response: Remember at all times that the service user is a person and not just a patient. They are not just a collection of signs and symptoms but a person with a life, family, interests and values. If the condition allows, ask them about themselves. What are their interests, hobbies? Show that you are interested in them as a person. You may be surprised just how amazing some patients' stories are! I have been privileged to hear first-hand accounts from Spitfire pilots who took part in the Battle of Britain. Talking to people puts them at ease and can, in some cases, distract them from what is happening at the time. Also, remember that non-verbal communication is just as important, if not more so, than what we say. Be aware of your body language and make eye contact.

Paramedic response: In addition to introductions, I try to place myself on the same level as a patient; this is particularly important with patients with dementia, as I'm trying to give them power over the situation with my non-verbal communication, thus making myself less of a threat.

The advice given in Box 9.2 may be useful if you find it quite difficult to instigate a conversation with your patient. Observing and reflecting on how other colleagues manage this will also be a useful approach to help you eventually develop your own style. Box 9.2 also demonstrates the importance of being patient-centred. There are both verbal and non-verbal communication strategies referred to by the contributors, all of which provide useful suggestions for the student paramedic.

c̃ Refer to Chapter 1 on the importance of transferable skills and communication.

As briefly discussed in Chapter 1, communication is highlighted as one of the six Cs of nursing, launched in 2012. Communication (and often the breakdown of it) is usually at the heart of NHS complaints and one reason why it has been placed at the top of the national agenda for nursing and subsequently other health-care professions.

The fundamentals of care: the six 6Cs

Initially focusing on nursing, the six Cs formed part of the National Nursing Strategy for England released in 2012. Since then, the NHS Commissioning Board has released operating instructions to all NHS staff to comply with the six Cs (Ford 2012). The six Cs are:

- Care
- Compassion
- Competence
- Communication
- Courage
- Commitment.

This will probably not be the last time you hear reference to these values, as it is recommended that these be embedded into teaching and learning, not only the clinical practice environment. Some of the explanation around each word is directly patient-focused and expressed in language that is clear to patients. For example, when explaining *communication* the quotation 'no decision about me without me' is used to describe what the ethos of communication should be for all NHS employees. It is recognised that communication is central to the success of caring relationships and to NHS teams working effectively together.

Sometimes communication breaks down. See the responses in Box 9.3.

Box 9.3 Can you give a brief account of a time when communication broke down and the consequences?

Paramedic mentor/PEd response: I found myself in an awful situation in a pub where we had been called to someone with a back injury. There was quite a large crowd and most people had been drinking. The lady with the back injury was flatly refusing to let me touch or treat her, whereas her friends were screaming at me to do something. Every attempt I made to help the patient was met with refusal, but her friends insisted I act against her will and just treat her. It was a no-win situation which became more and more heated. By the end, communication had totally broken down and sadly the police had to be called.

:🚨: **Paramedic mentor/PEd response:** I was working solo on a rapid response vehicle and attended a road traffic collision where a female had come off of her push bike. It was immediately obvious that this lady was critically unwell and I required more kit than I had immediately available to me once I got out the car. I utilised members of the public and the police to get kit from my car, and this meant I needed to give them my keys. When they returned the keys I put them into a bag beside me, rather than keeping them on my person. Once the crew arrived I travelled with the patient and left the other member of staff with my car, telling them the keys were in the bag. Unfortunately the member of staff couldn't find the keys and started asking others left on scene if they knew what I had done with them. While I was on a five-mile journey with the patient, the story developed, like Chinese whispers, into the fact that I had given my keys to an off-duty police officer and they had gone missing!

The consequences of this were that: the police investigated someone impersonating a police officer (as they knew there was not an off-duty officer on scene); a fleet manager was dispatched from 30 miles away with a spare set of keys (the keys were in the bag throughout); and the car remained unlocked, posing a safety risk.

I learnt from this situation that had I communicated effectively before I left the scene and ensured the keys had been found, the above sequence of events wouldn't have occurred. It is extremely easy in busy situations for communications to be misheard or for the initial meaning to change throughout. Unfortunately, this can lead to negative outcomes.

The contributors' responses in Box 9.3 show how easy it is for communication breakdown to occur. When it does, it can lead to a series of events which are sometimes avoidable, other times not, but are always uncomfortable. Communication is central to your role as a professional and needs to be afforded respect and be practised, reflected upon and continually improved, even once you are a registered paramedic.

The other Cs are also important:

- *Care.* NHS England (2012) makes it clear that care is the core business of the NHS and that care defines who we are and our work. Our patients should therefore expect that the care we deliver is consistently right for them.

- *Compassion.* Relationships between patients and NHS employees should involve not only compassion but also empathy, respect and dignity when providing care to patients.
- *Competence.* All people in a caring role must be competent to understand an individual's health and social care needs. It is having 'the expertise, clinical and technical knowledge to deliver care based on research and evidence'.
- *Commitment.* This refers to our responsibility to our patients and the fact we need to build on our commitment to improve care and patient experiences.
- *Courage.* Staff should be enabled to 'do the right thing for the people we care for, to speak up when we have concerns'. An alternative word for this would be asking NHS staff to *advocate* for their patients.

The one C that may appear to be slightly out of place is that of courage. Remember that the six Cs were developed at a time when there were significant failings being reported in parts of the NHS. The inquiry that led to the Francis Report (Department of Health 2013a) was under way, and this was to find that NHS employees knew care standards were not as they should be but failed to get their concerns heard satisfactorily.

CASE STUDY 9.1 THE JOYS AND DIFFICULTIES OF ADVOCATING FOR A PATIENT?

I handed over a lady with severe asthma to ED. She was agitated and clearly hypoxic. The staff took the handover, but did not accept my explanation of how seriously ill I thought she was. I was so worried that I found the person in charge of the department and voiced my concerns. She assessed the patient and agreed with me, called an anaesthetist, and the patient was sedated and admitted to the intensive care unit. If I hadn't done this for my patient, I am sure she would have gone into respiratory arrest.

It isn't always easy to act as an advocate for a patient, but remember that sometimes you may be the only voice they have. If this were your mother or father, wouldn't you want someone to speak up for them and safeguard their best interests? I know I would! For that reason, I have never shied away from this, no matter how difficult it has sometimes been. It is particularly difficult when acting as an advocate for a patient involves a colleague and I don't underestimate just how hard this can be. All I will say is that most reasonable people know in their heart of hearts when something is wrong and, as a paramedic there to care for those sick or vulnerable, it is your duty to speak out.

Advocacy is a crucial aspect of our role as professionals. As Case Study 9.1 demonstrates, sometimes it is easier to advocate on behalf of your patient than it is to speak up for yourself. Your uniform also generally empowers you to speak on behalf of your patient. It may save someone's life one day.

Current issues within the care professions

It is clear that the NHS is under intense scrutiny and will continue to remain so. One thing that you need to be clear about is that your working environment, the NHS, is subject to almost constant change as a result of vacillating political agendas and policies, as the comments in Box 9.4 highlight.

Any clinician who makes a point of being up to date with health-care agendas is in a prime position to make the most of any new initiatives, innovations and education available to them. Initially this may be of interest from a personal development perspective (as the comments in Box 9.4 explain), but eventually an interest in the health-care agenda of today will positively impact on the care provided to patients.

Although fundamentally investigating and referring to hospital-based care and patients' experiences of care, the Francis Report (Department of Health 2013a) will be highlighted here. The Francis Inquiry examined 1 million pages of evidence, heard from 250 witnesses, had 139 days of oral hearings, produced a 1700-page report with 290 recommendations, and cost £13 million. As a consequence of the extensive and intense report that resulted, the recommendations made by the government are extensive and a significant challenge for NHS trusts to implement. As a student paramedic, you will witness some of the changes that are a

Box 9.4 Is it worth keeping up to date with the most recent health-care agendas? Why?

Paramedic response: Throughout my studies the emphasis on keeping up to date with health-care initiatives was reinforced. While studying I didn't really understand the value, but some of the new roles being created in my trust have developed out of the national agenda and demand. I have kept a close eye on this since registration and have undertaken modules/study days that have kept me up to date, and this led to me securing a place on one of the first courses to enable me to practise in an advanced role and try to keep people in their own homes as far as possible. Had I not foreseen this development, I would not have been able to put myself in the position to be one of the first to be educated for this new and exciting role.

Academic response: It is vital to keep up to date with the most recent health-care agendas, as ultimately many of them will impact directly upon our practice. This does not just relate to clinical updates, but to the many and varied roles being created in the ambulance service and the evolving scope of practice. Policies impact upon fundamentals, such as what the role of a paramedic will be in the future and what areas must be covered in the curriculum as a result of this. By having an awareness of where the profession is heading due to health-care agendas we can keep one step ahead and ensure we are prepared when changes are implemented.

result of the Francis Report, as they are not only confined to hospital systems.

The government's initial response to the Francis Inquiry, a report titled *Patients First and Foremost* (Department of Health 2013b), took the form of a five-point plan:

- Preventing problems
- Detecting problems quickly
- Taking action promptly
- Ensuring robust accountability
- Ensuring staff are trained and motivated.

As you can see, these points can be applied to any NHS trust, not just hospital services. One of the keys to achieving and maintaining the above five points is the strength and development of clinical leadership (Blaber and Harris 2014).

This chapter has served to introduce some of the current main political drivers in the care professions and includes some specific information regarding your interactions with patients and their families.

Suggested reading

Blaber, A.Y. and Harris, G. (2014) *Clinical Leadership for Paramedics*. Maidenhead: Open University Press.

Department of Health (2013a) *Report of the Mid Staffordshire NHS Foundation Trust Public Inquiry: Executive Summary*. London: The Stationery Office.

Department of Health (2013b) *Patients First and Foremost: The Initial Government Response to the Report of the Mid Staffordshire NHS Foundation Trust Public Inquiry*. London: Department of Health.

Ford, S. (2012) All NHS staff told to embrace nursing's '6Cs'. *Nursing Times*, 18 December. Available at: http://www.nursingtimes.net/nursing-practice/ specialisms/management/all-nhs-staff-told-to-embrace-nursings-6cs/ 5053011.article (accessed 15 September 2014).

NHS England (2012) *Our Culture of Compassionate Care*. London: NHS England. Available at: http://www.england.nhs.uk/wp-content/uploads/ 2012/12/6c-a5-leaflet.pdf (accessed 18 January 2015).

10 WHAT SUPPORT IS THERE WHEN ON PLACEMENT?

This chapter will outline who is there to help you when you need support and will give examples of ways you can contact them. One key message is to make use of the resources available and talk to those who are equipped to support you.

There are formal support strategies for all undergraduate health-care students. For student paramedics the HCPC (2014) has a specific section in its *Standards of Education and Training* (SETs) document relating to practice placements. Table 10.1 highlights the SETs that are relevant to the support available while on placement.

The detail provided in Table 10.1 will enable you to appreciate that your time spent in clinical placement is carefully guided and planned. It is monitored by the HCPC and reviewed as part of the annual monitoring process undertaken by the HEI and HCPC. Before student paramedics can go on placement, a lot of preparatory work is undertaken by both the HEI and the ambulance trust. Placements require auditing and staff may need educating, in order to act as effective, supportive paramedic educators (PEds). In the same way that you should not embark on this career lightly, your HEI and ambulance trust are taking your welfare, education and support needs seriously.

The term 'PPEd' or 'PEd' is specific to paramedic education, but in some localities the term 'mentor' is also being used on paramedic programmes. Also, when you attend non-ambulance placements you may be supported by a qualified mentor. Mentors are registered professionals who have undergone a further period of education and gained a mentorship qualification in order that they can ably support students who come to their clinical area, whether they are nurses, midwives or community staff, for example. For the purposes of this chapter, the focus will be specifically on the student paramedic in ambulance placements and the role of the people who will be responsible for supporting you.

Table 10.1 SETs relating to support on practice placement (HCPC 2014)

SET number	
5.3	The practice placement settings must provide a safe and supportive environment.
5.7	Practice placement educators [PPEds] must have relevant knowledge, skills and experience.
5.8	Practice placement educators must undertake appropriate practice placement educator training.
5.9	Practice placement educators must be appropriately registered, unless other arrangements are agreed.
5.11	Students, practice placement providers and practice placement educators must be fully prepared for placement which will include information about an understanding of: • the learning outcomes to be achieved; • the timings and the duration of any placement experience and associated records to be maintained; • expectations of professional conduct; • the assessment procedures including the implications of, and any action to be taken in the case of, failure to progress; and • communication and lines of responsibility.

Reflection: points to consider

Think about the programmes that you have investigated to date or your own programme if you are already studying to become a paramedic. Can you list the support available from:

● The university perspective?
● Clinical practice?

Mentor/paramedic educator

The following student comments speak for themselves and really highlight the value of mentor/PEd support in the journey of the student paramedic.

Student paramedic comment: I had some amazing mentors during my ambulance placements. In fact everyone at both stations was really friendly and keen to help me develop. Any time I heard someone talk about 'students' it was during some friendly banter which just reinforced the fact that I was considered one of the team.

My PEd/mentors were very supportive. They did more than simply allow me to watch them or occasionally let me mop a patient's brow. They encouraged me to get involved with clinical procedures and patient care (often when they felt I was ready but I wasn't so sure).

They had a confidence in me that helped me to develop as a student. We would debrief after most jobs and talk about what we could have done differently. This was often a two-way conversation; my mentors were always ready to learn from me if I had a good suggestion or some insight from a recent lecture.

Student paramedic comment: Studying, whether for 2 or 3 years, can be challenging enough. With paramedic studies you follow the typical university structure of lectures and increasing levels of writing, but you are also thrown in the deep end of a career that you may have very little real knowledge of. This is where your PEd takes you by the hand and guides you through all your questions and eases your fears – or so you hope. This turned out to be the biggest challenge for me, while year 1 is generally recommended to be a *viewing* rather than *doing* year, it is still a time where you need that extra boost of confidence from those you will be attending in front of in the coming year. The first year goes by so fast, there is no time to lose. I had a poor experience with a PEd whose personality vastly differed from my own, who could not understand the way I worked (or learned) best and soon enough gave up on me. This continued into year 2. So before I knew it, I was in year 3, with the pressure on to perform. Unsurprisingly, my confidence took a knock and almost led me to believe I was not right for the job. All because one person got the wrong impression of me, based on their own opinion of who they thought I should have been, or the level I should have been at rather than referring to the practice documentation.

Building relationships throughout placement, finding just one person who shares similar personality style and teaching qualities, or who at least respects your learning style, can be the difference between you just ticking boxes on placement and really experiencing in the moment, using it to your full potential. With the help of my university and a great previous mentor who I confided in, my confidence slowly grew. Being shown respect as a colleague rather than a student makes all the difference. There are plenty of 'big' characters, as there are anywhere. Some you will work well with and others you will try to work well with, but you will not be able to impress everyone while practising as a paramedic, let alone as a student.

As can be seen from these experiences relating to PEds, the role is central to the student paramedic's development of confidence and competence. The PEd role, as identified by the College of Paramedics (2014: 47) is 'extremely important and comes with significant responsibility. The actions and examples set by the paramedic educator during clinical placements have lasting consequences, which include positive and negative influences.' These points are echoed by the student paramedic comments above, where the reality of the positive and negative consequences is clearly articulated. Case Study 10.1 presents one student's experience of being mentored in more detail.

CASE STUDY 10.1

During my first year undertaking my paramedic studies I got to know and worked with my mentor/PEd – all was well. I also felt I got to know other staff across the course of the year. I really enjoyed it, felt I was learning and progressing well.

At the beginning of my second year I returned to station to find my mentor had left. I was assigned a new mentor, and over the course of several weeks, it became clear that we were very different personalities and did not like each other. The way my new mentor worked was very different from what I had experienced in year 1. My mentor/PEd began to see less and less of me, I felt unsupported, lacked direction, confidence and felt my progress stalling. Some of the other clinicians I had come to know well in my previous year had also left the station. I began to dread going to placement, and this must have showed when I was there. I was not my usual enthusiastic self.

At the end of the year I bumped into my year 1 mentor/PEd by accident. There were a few other issues too, but the end result was that my original mentor offered to mentor me until the end of my programme and this was agreed by the university team too. I finished my practice experience feeling confident and positive, very different to how I felt in year 2.

My mentor/PEd always told me there was no doubt I would make a great paramedic, the only thing I needed was self-confidence. When I started my new first job as a paramedic, my mentor told me I could contact him any time if I felt I needed it. We still remain in contact – now years after registration.

I had some negative experiences on my placements but the positives outweighed these. As well as my mentor I have other members of staff to thank for making me welcome, part of the team, and also my programme leader and personal tutor, who always made time for me.

Placement is rarely without issues, as Case Study 10.1 describes. The importance of your mentor/PEd is well illustrated by the case study and other comments. Other staff on station are also part of the student's support mechanism, whether they are mentors/PEds or not. On-station staff are the staff who work at the ambulance station, such as technicians or support worker grade staff. Their involvement is central to the student's experience and development. There are a variety of other people in roles which are designed and intended to be supportive and useful to student paramedics.

Link lecturers, lecturer practitioners and associate lecturers

Other titles that you may come across are those of link lecturer, lecturer practitioner and associate lecturer. They are different roles, but may also mean different things in different geographical areas. See Box 10.1 for different terminology relating to the roles; it is important that you become familiar with the terminology used in your programme.

Box 10.1 Can you provide the definition of 'link lecturer' in your location/area?

🎓 **Academic response:** 'Link lecturer' refers to a named university member of staff who is linked to a specific ambulance station/area. This person should be the first port of call for any employee, PEd or student paramedic if they are having difficulties, problems, issues in placement. This named person would also be responsible for auditing the placement area and providing feedback from student and PEd evaluations after students complete their placements.

🎓 **Academic response:** In some localities, the link lecturer can also be called an 'academic advisor' or 'academic mentor'. This is a named member of the university staff who will have had students allocated to him/her and will be the first port of call for their students should they experience any problems or need any help. Your link lecturer may visit you on placement from time to time making sure that everything is running smoothly. Placements are audited and generally managed by a placements lead who will also oversee the link lecturers and allocate students to them. Students find it valuable to have a named person they can go to if they need anything rather than randomly asking a member of the academic team if they need anything.

🎓 **Academic response:** In our university, link lecturers are referred to as 'zone tutors'. A zone tutor is a member of the paramedic teaching team who is allocated a practice area and provides an important link between the practice setting and the university programme team. The practice mentor and the academic zone tutor are jointly responsible for students who are on placement in their allocated area. The academic zone tutor has many roles, including providing support for practice mentors and students alike during their placement, and briefing and debriefing students before and after placements.

Can you provide the definition of 'lecturer practitioner' in your location/area?

🎓 **Academic response:** A lecturer practitioner (LP) is a paramedic who works some of the time in practice as a paramedic and some of the time in the university teaching and supporting student paramedics on academic courses. The LP role may also include supporting PEd/mentors in practice and potentially visiting students in clinical placement occasionally.

🎓 **Academic response:** Lecturer practitioners can also be known as 'associate lecturers'. These are staff who still work in practice but who also come in to the university to teach or assist with practical modules. Many are also on-road mentors.

As with many of the other aspects in previous chapters, refer to the university programme handbook where there may be a glossary of terms, flowchart or description of the roles of the staff involved in delivery and support of your studies.

Academic support

The staff supporting you will be registered health-care professionals. In most cases your programme will consist of a mixture of paramedics and other health-care professionals who will have relevant experience and expertise in the areas they are asked to teach you.

Student paramedic comment: Our lecturers were very good at supporting us academically. I don't think I ever got through all the suggested reading, links to videos of clinical procedures and extra resources, etc. that they all made available to us along with their lectures. They were also available to see if you had a problem or questions about some piece of work you were struggling with. Obviously, they had a vested interest in seeing us do well, but I'd say they were genuinely pleased for us when we achieved things we had been aiming for.

If something cropped up on placement – like a traumatic job – our uni lecturers would hear about it and get in touch to check we were all right. When I went to a job which was potentially upsetting for a 'fresh out of the box' first-year I found an email from one of my lecturers waiting for me when I arrived home from shift asking if I was OK.

As you will note from the above comments and Box 10.2, on the whole, academics recognise the demands of the student paramedic role. The support is readily available, if you want it. Student paramedics need to remember that their academic staff are also caring professionals. This caring tendency may be experienced by students who undergo difficult times during their studies. It may be that your academic staff feel you need more specialist help and they will be able to help you access this via the university systems and processes.

🔗 Refer to Chapter 5 for more information on learning support.

Box 10.2 What would your message to student paramedics be about accessing academic support?

🎓 **Academic response:** Talk to your academic staff – we are not mind-readers. We are here to help, with anything really, but if you do not talk to us, how do you expect us to know you are struggling? It may be a new issue for you, or something you find difficult to talk about, but it is unlikely to be something we have not come across before. Find a way to tell us, write a note/email if you feel you cannot talk to us face to face initially. Ask a friend to help you. Just approach any member of academic staff that you feel comfortable with, it does not even need to be a member of your programme team. Use the university support system; maybe they can support you in speaking to your academic staff. Be brave and we will try our best to advise and help you.

🎓 **Academic response:** Whilst it is in our interest that you do well and have a good experience both in university and on placement, it goes far deeper than this. I am genuinely thrilled to see my students develop, gain confidence and achieve. My students are part of my 'paramedic family' and I am there to support and look after them wherever I can. A lot of staff feel the same way, so never be reticent about approaching us for help. Some of the time we may know you need help with something before you do!

Academic support is available to you, but, as has been mentioned in other chapters, a variety of support is given to you by your friends, families, other members of your cohort and previous cohorts. If this is the route you choose to take, make sure the advice you are being given is accurate, correct and not misleading. If you are in any doubt about this, contact someone from your academic team to ensure you have the most up-to-date information available. Your colleagues may have very good intentions, but what applied to their cohort may not be the same for your group.

Debrief

The debrief is a way of discussing and reflecting on practice issues. It can be undertaken in a formal or informal way; it may often be a two-way conversation with your mentor/PEd. However it is carried out, the effectiveness and educational benefits of the debrief should not be underestimated, as Box 10.3 explains.

⌀ Refer to the introductory discussion on reflection in Chapter 3.

Box 10.3 Can you provide a brief example of a formal or informal debrief you were involved in and how it helped you, or not?

📖 **Student paramedic response:** I went to a particularly nasty resus in the second year. The patient had a terminal illness but had not signed a do not attempt resuscitation (DNAR) form. The crew I was with were unsure about whether to attempt CPR or not, but decided to go ahead. The resus attempt was particularly traumatic for us due to the nature of the patient's condition (fortunately, the patient's family were not in the room). A paramedic arrived to back us up, but we were unable to resuscitate the patient. Afterwards we had an informal debrief with the paramedic, who clarified that where a patient is in the end stages of a terminal illness and there are clear indications in their patient notes that they will shortly die (and in this case a close relative who could confirm the patient intended to sign a DNAR), we would have been justified in not attempting to resuscitate. This meant we could have spared the patient and ourselves a significantly harrowing experience. The debrief prompted me to study and clarify the law, local policy and expectations upon us as paramedics, in respect of performing CPR on patients with a terminal illness, so that I might act in the best interest of any future patient and in the best interest of my own future mental health.

Important point: Also of particular importance here is the local ambulance service NHS trust's policy on end-of-life care and resuscitation.

:🚨: **Paramedic mentor/PEd response:** I have always found informal debriefs more helpful than formal ones. This is just my opinion, but I have found that things feel less pressured when informal measures can be taken to address issues that have arisen needing a debrief. Debriefs are useful after an upsetting incident, whether an incident that did not go so well or one that went like clockwork.

It is important that you also ask to have a formal or informal discussion with someone, to help you reflect on any incident that may have worried you. On occasions, mentors/PEds can forget that you are a student and do not consider that the calls you have been to that day are anything out of the ordinary. But, for example, you may not have seen a person who has died before – this will affect you, but may not be something that your mentor/PEd would usually debrief. The same adage applies: 'if you do not tell us, we do not know!'

CASE STUDIES 10.2

Informal 'hot' debrief
Following a road traffic collision in rush hour in a busy town, where a single patient sustained significant injuries and consequently received a rapid sequence intubation and a finger thoracotomy pre-hospitally, a 'hot' debrief was conducted by the lead clinician outside the ED. Initial concerns, thoughts and feelings were discussed, and I felt happy with the sequence of events and had no underlying concerns. However, this was in essence the end of the incident as far as others were concerned. As days progressed and after I had time to reflect, I had questions which were difficult to find answers to, as the people involved in the incident weren't immediately available. The hot debrief meant that I was not affected emotionally and my questions were purely from an education and interest perspective.

Informal 'hot' debrief followed by formal planned
multi-professional debrief
I attended a paediatric cardiac arrest; this understandably was a highly emotive situation. It occurred at the end of my shift, the circumstances of the incident were complex and there was an awful

lot of adrenaline flowing through me at the time of the hot debrief. For all concerned our thinking may not have been clear, objective or logical at the time of the hot debrief. I went home and did my own reflection and review of the emergency. Colleagues and staff provided me with support over the next few days while a planned multi-professional debrief was being organised. The planned debrief occurred 10 days later and included everybody from all disciplines involved in the event. This gave us the opportunity to discuss the whole event from the initial 999 call through to the toxicology and scan results. Thorough discussion occurred and a detailed and full understanding was obtained. Wider perspectives were discussed and that enabled me to appreciate a more holistic view of the event. It enabled me to bring the event to a close.

In my opinion, the combination of a hot debrief at the time and a following planned debrief was the best outcome and the best solution, enabling closure to highly distressing and emotive incidents.

Formal debriefs in the ambulance service usually occur after specific untoward incidents, such as large-scale accidents. These events will be organised, involve various levels of staff, managerial staff and specialist staff, such as counsellors and therapists. It is highly possible that the student paramedic is overlooked, not through any malice but as these events are triggered by internal systems that may not automatically include student paramedics. By keeping in contact with your mentor/PEd, you should be able to participate in any such event and may be given time away from university to take part.

✐ Refer to Chapter 12 for more on difficult cases and Chapter 13 for more on resilience.

Colleagues, friends and family

As a student paramedic, you will come to recognise the importance of the support available to you from colleagues, friends and family.

Student paramedic comment: At first you tell everyone everything that you've seen and done as you are just excited about being 'out there' whizzing around in a yellow truck! But as time goes on, I started to go into less and less detail about jobs with family and friends. Partly as I wanted to protect family from some of the things we see but also because I found a few friends just wanted to hear 'horror stories' – one friend wanted to know 'what's the worst thing you've seen this week?' every time I saw him. I didn't want the story of a patient's suffering to be a source of pleasure for someone else, so I would say we hadn't been to any eventful jobs, even if we had. And there is confidentiality to seriously consider.

As students, we would lean on each other for support a lot as well as our mentors and uni staff. This was because these were all people who had a greater understanding of the work we were involved with and could sympathise, not merely empathise.

One of the support structures on placement is humour. There is a definite 'ambulance humour', which can be quite dark at times. It's used as a coping strategy against stress and it tends to work. However, it is an 'acquired' thing. At first some fellow students were quite shocked to hear some of the jokes that are made in the crew room, only to find themselves cracking the same sort of jokes a few months later when the reality of the job had begun to kick in. Things like this draw you closer together as a team but also build a separation towards some aspects of the job between you and your folks outside. I guess you learn to go to different people depending on what type of support you need.

The student comment above relates to a variety of coping mechanisms and the fact that this changes as time progresses, as your professionalism develops and as your appreciation of the seriousness of the situations you are witnessing deepens. You may also develop a protective mechanism towards your close family and friends, not wishing to compromise confidentiality or bother them with your worries or concerns. As the student mentions, the style of humour used in the ambulance service and emergency services generally can be quite a shock for people hearing it the first time. It serves a purpose, but should be used with caution, depending on the situation, your location and people accompanying you. As a student paramedic you may witness humour from your practice colleagues, mentors/PEds, but your mentor/PEd may deem it inappropriate for you, the student, to be the person making the jokes. 'Double standards' perhaps, but they may want you to earn your rite of passage in order to use the humour eventually. Learn to act with professionalism at all times before you get to this point.

This chapter has examined the various types of support available to you generally and specifically while you are on placement. In discussing this, it is important to mention the value of debriefing incidents that may affect you, however little or large they seem to you. The message is: keep talking.

Suggested reading

College of Paramedics (2014) *Paramedic Curriculum Guidance* (3rd edn). Bridgwater: College of Paramedics. Available at: https://www. collegeofparamedics.co.uk/downloads/Curriculum_Guidance_2014.pdf (accessed 18 February 2005).

Health and Care Professions Council (2014) *Standards of Education and Training*. London: HCPC. Available at: http://www.hcpc-uk.org.uk/aboutregistration/standards/sets/index.asp (accessed 18 January 2015).

Read your programme handbook for more information on the roles of clinicians involved with your programme. Familiarise yourself with the titles used and the differences in the roles.

Read any policies of your ambulance trust related to incident debrief, and speak to someone at the trust if you need to, so that you are aware of the processes involved in both formal and informal debriefs in the clinical environment.

11 ASSESSMENT IN PRACTICE

All HEI health-care programmes include assessment of students in the clinical environment. The assessment process varies from institution to institution, but fundamentally it involves skills, attitudes, behaviours and competencies being assessed by a registered professional over a period of time. Usually the assessment is allocated academic credits, and therefore forms part of a module/unit. In some institutions the assessment of practice is graded, in other institutions the student is assessed and is passed or failed. This is not as drastic as it sounds, as this chapter will explain.

How are you assessed in practice?

Your mentors/PEds and a myriad of other ambulance staff are assessing you whenever you are in the practice environment. As the College of Paramedics (2014: 42) suggests, a 'range of . . . supervising and assessment methods that promote an integrated approach of theory and practice should be employed'. The suggestion is that students' assessment in practice should include:

- Encouraging students to adopt critical thinking approaches to patient care
- Encouraging independent learning through reflective practice
- Promoting and assessing professional conduct
- Employing evidence-based practice
- Appreciating the importance of audit and research.

Most institutions will require your mentors/PEds to assess you while you are working in the clinical area. How this is achieved, the people involved and the documentation used will vary from institution to institution. Generally, though, you will need to document events in practice, and provide signatures from your mentor/PEd in a formal assessment document that (in line with theoretical work) needs to be submitted to the university on a certain date for analysis.

Who assesses you in practice?

Usually it is your named mentor/PEd who is responsible for teaching you, supporting you and also assessing you in the clinical environment. These are diverse roles and are one reason why paramedics who want to become mentors/PEds require additional educational training and support. It can be difficult for both student and mentor/PEd to balance the roles and responsibilities they each have and to get things right all of the time. As the paramedic/PEd response in Box 11.1 shows, the role is not only one of assessment.

Box 11.1 What have you found is the best way of dealing with the fact that your PEd is also the person assessing you in practice? Does that create any issues? If so, what?

📖 **Student response:** Initially there is pressure to impress, but being yourself is important. The more you relax, the easier the process will become. On one occasion I did have one of my mentors refusing to pass me. The PEd kept going back over one incident; it was a one-off and never happened again. The assessment should be over a period of time and not representative of one specific issue/incident that never occurred again. This was frustrating, but was my only bad experience.

👮 **Paramedic/PEd response:** Initially you may feel you are under constant scrutiny from your mentor. Hopefully, as time goes on and you get to know your mentor, this will feel less and less the case. Although you are being assessed you are also becoming a part of that ambulance crew and you will work together as a team. Just concentrate on your patients and your job. Your mentor is there not only to assess you, but also to teach and advise.

As alluded to in Box 11.1, there are a vast array of areas, not just skills, being assessed. Your personal behaviour, professional actions, ability to work as part of a team and, of course, communication skills are a few of the many areas that your mentor/PEd will be taking note of during your time with them. Assessment can be both formal and informal in nature.

Formal and informal assessment

Expect your mentor/PEd to use both formal and informal approaches to assessment. Even if you are not working with your mentor/PEd, they will ask their colleagues about your progress. Whilst ambulance staff will do their best to help you feel at home and happy in the environment, you will be under scrutiny – however, it will not feel this way. Your continued exposure to the clinical environment, in many cases, will form part of your informal assessment. All mentors/PEds, as individuals, work differently, and you will have the opportunity to discuss this with them. As the student comment below explains, it is not only about your ability to perform individual skills.

> **Student paramedic comment:** Assessment in practice is also about how you present yourself, your communication skills, and manner. A paramedic is more than just a person who knows how to take basic patient observations.

How you present yourself and your manner is not something that can be assessed on one occasion, it is an ongoing informal assessment by your mentors/PEd about your suitability for the professional role. It should be continually assessed over a period of time.

Formative and summative assessments

There are occasions when your assessment does not count towards your final grade, and others when the assessment is more formal (see the definitions box).

> **Definitions: Formative and summative**
>
> There are two words that are commonly used in respect of assessment of practice:
>
> *Formative* refers to the opportunity to practise. This can relate to academic work or clinical skills. You may be given the opportunity to submit a formative piece of work, you will receive feedback on your

efforts, but it will not be given a mark or grade. The same applies to clinical skills and the opportunity to practise them and be given feedback on your progress. The intention is that you act on the feedback provided (either written or verbal) in order to improve your academic work or clinical performance.

Summative refers to a more formal assessment. Some academic work will require you to submit it for summative assessment. This work will be given a mark or grade, and you will receive written feedback on your efforts. In some cases academic work and clinical skills may only be summatively assessed as pass or fail.

Discuss this with your programme team for further clarification, if you are unsure about these terms.

How best to carry out summative assessments is a decision for the mentor/ PEd; this decision is sometimes made in conjunction with the student. The opportunistic nature of paramedic practice means that formal summative assessments are rarely possible to plan. Usually the procedure or skill will have been formatively assessed by the mentor/PEd on the several previous occasions you have demonstrated the procedure (under supervision). Consequently, your mentor/PEd is happy to pass you summatively on the next occasion that you encounter the same procedure/skill. As you can see by the student's comment below, it is not the case that once you have passed the procedure/skill you will always perform it perfectly every time.

Student paramedic comment: Don't worry if you get things wrong – you're a student, and your mentor is there to ensure you don't make any serious mistakes. It is an old cliché, but it's true that you learn more from your mistakes than your successes. I had been passed summatively by my mentor on the skill of cannulation. But, one time I forgot to release the tourniquet after cannulating a patient. Their hand was going purple. My mentor reminded me and said afterwards, 'don't worry about it, now you've made that mistake you'll never do it again – it's a learning curve'. The fact is, I've never left a tourniquet on a patient since.

The learning process, as explained by the student's experience above, is one that has ups and downs. If, however, the student had continued to leave the tourniquet on the patient for too long a period of time, after every cannulation performed, the mentor/PEd would have needed to review their decision about the student being competent at the skill of cannulation.

It may be the case that you have met a certain skill only a couple of times during the time you have spent with your mentor/PEd. Imagine that the deadline to submit your practice document may be looming and you need to be summatively assessed. Your mentor/PEd may decide to be creative and utilise simulation within the practice environment. This will enable your mentor/PEd to test your accomplishment of skill competence, test your underpinning theoretical knowledge and your professional behaviour. However, it is crucial that the vast majority of your assessment of practice should take place with patients and not in a simulated environment. Simulated assessments are a compromise and can be used to enable your mentor/PEd to fully complete your documentation and may also enable them to provide some additional structured teaching. Many students experience simulations that are additional learning opportunities, organised by their mentor/PEd team in the practice environment.

⌀ Refer to Chapter 6 for more detail on simulation.

What do I do if I don't get on with my mentor/PEd?

As with any situation, people sometimes do not get on, personalities clash, but they still have to work together. You are preparing to work as a professional and, as such, this entails having to work with people you may prefer not to work with. Of course it makes things easier if everyone on the vehicle gets along well as a team, but this does not mean you are anything more than colleagues. Many people work alongside each other in a professional capacity and work well in a team, but may not choose to be friends outside the working environment. Mentors/PEds should keep a professional distance from students, as on occasions it may be necessary to fail a student in practice, and this is made more difficult if friendships are involved. Conversely, the student may not be happy with a mentor/PEd's action or decision, and friendships may make this situation more difficult to report and manage for the student paramedic.

Following on from the previous paragraph, on some occasions people may act unprofessionally and it may be necessary to hold discussions between practice staff, the student and university staff, if in the first instance the issues cannot be solved by the student and paramedic mentor/ PEd. Case Study 10.1 in the previous chapter describes the student's perspective on some of the consequences of student–mentor relationship breakdown and also the value of mentor/PEd support. If after employing numerous different strategies, the situation is not improving for all parties, it may be wise to recognise each other's differences. On rare occasions, the student paramedic may find themselves moved to a different area or may request to be relocated, if the issues and problems encountered are insurmountable. The vast majority of student experiences in practice working alongside a mentor/PEd and other ambulance staff are positive in nature. Students report that it is here that their learning, support and personal development are fostered and encouraged.

As with any theoretical work, you need to be fully aware of what is required of you. Assessment of practice is no different. Take the documentation/work required seriously, read any handbooks or instructions that are provided for you. Ensure you are clear on your responsibilities and at an early opportunity discuss the assessment process with your mentor/PEd. This should enable you both to have a clear vision of how the time spent together should progress and will clarify roles and responsibilities.

Suggested reading

College of Paramedics (2014) *Paramedic Curriculum Guidance* (3rd edn). Bridgwater: College of Paramedics. Available at: https://www. collegeofparamedics.co.uk/downloads/Curriculum_Guidance_2014.pdf (accessed 18 February 2005).

Barrett, K. and Nelson, L. (2014) Mentorship and preceptorship. In A.Y. Blaber and G. Harris (eds.) *Clinical Leadership for Paramedics*. Maidenhead: Open University Press.

Read your university and practice assessment handbooks relating to practice and the roles/responsibilities of both the student and mentor/PEd.

12 DIFFICULT CASES

During the course of your studies you will care for an immense variety of individuals under an immense variety of circumstances. Some cases will inevitably be difficult.

What types of situation might you find yourself in?

You may find yourself in any situation! The variety of the paramedic role is probably one of the aspects that initially attracted you to the role. The student paramedic comments below describe the range of situations experienced and some of their effects.

> **Student paramedic comments:** I've been to all types of situations, from patients high on drugs waving knives at the police, to a lady who wanted us to wipe her elderly mother's bottom after she'd been to the toilet.
>
> I found I wasn't affected by the jobs I thought I would be. It was often the non-trauma jobs, where people had reached a point of real distress, which stayed with me after the event. You find yourself thinking about them weeks later, hoping that patient is doing OK. Due to patient confidentiality and data protection you can't find out what happened to a patient after you handed them over at hospital. Sometimes not knowing what happened next is difficult. You have to develop a professional distance and protect yourself from letting things get to you.
>
> It is not easy, balancing compassion and concern for others with keeping a healthy distance. I found my mentor was the best person to talk to as he knew what a balancing act this can be and seemed to have found a way of doing it.

Students often expect the more dramatic, large-scale events, such as road traffic collisions, to affect them most. This might be the case, but as the student paramedic comments demonstrate, often smaller-scale, more personal situations are equally powerful.

You may have a certain amount of preparation time when you are en route to a call, and this is psychologically extremely valuable, but there is always the element of surprise, as Case Study 12.1 describes.

CASE STUDY 12.1

It can be very challenging to have psychologically prepared yourself to attend a particular type of incident due to information given by control and find yourself faced with something very different. When I was still an ambulance technician we were called to an 80-year-old lady who had fallen in the early hours of the morning. As we travelled to the job over a large flyover we came across a double fatal RTC involving two motorcyclists, a van and an HGV. Because I was psychologically prepared for going to the patient who had had a fall it took me a few moments to process what I was seeing in front of me. I have heard many paramedics say the same thing when they have expected to attend an adult patient and found a child, etc.

Additionally, it may be the most surprising jobs that you find have affected you. Being able to strongly identify with a patient may mean you are more affected by an incident. Do not feel guilty if a job has not affected you in the way you feel it should. Just because something affects one person in a particular way does not mean it will affect another the same. Different things affect different people in different ways and it can be very hard to predict what these will be or how they will affect you.

The following section describes in more detail the potential for situations to arouse feelings, or the surprising lack of feelings, alluded to in Case Study 12.1. As individuals and professionals, we will experience a range of emotions when caring for our patients and families.

How might this make you feel?

Consider the reflection points below before reading on.

Reflection: points to consider

Think about a difficult time for you personally.

What emotions did you experience? List them.

The contributors below have been very honest and open in their discussion of their emotions and feelings. There is little commentary to add to their powerful explanation of some situations and subsequent emotions/ feelings they have experienced.

Box 12.1 Reflect on a difficult case. Can you describe your emotions and feelings?

📖 **Student paramedic response:** I went to a lady who had taken a big overdose and had tried to hide herself in the woods. She was found by some people walking their dog. When we got there she was semi-conscious and couldn't speak, but still tried to resist any help.

I had to look through the patient's handbag for any medications and identity. In her bag was the suicide note she had written. It struck me that I was the first person to read it and that if she died I would be the first person to pass on the information she wanted to leave behind; that made me feel really strange for quite a while after the event.

We got the patient to hospital, but after that I don't know what happened to her. I don't know if it's odd, but it struck me that when someone leaves a suicide note they are trusting that the person who finds it will act as the link between them and those they wrote it to. I know other paramedics think nothing of it, but I feel there's something special about that.

Different jobs create different feelings, not always the same as those of your colleagues. Reflecting on a job and your feelings towards it helps make sense of the whole thing, putting it into a context that makes it easier to handle.

🕯 **Paramedic mentor/PEd response:** I attended a sudden unexpected cardiac arrest of a relatively young gentleman who collapsed in front of his wife and young family. Although all efforts were made to revive this gentleman, we were unable to.

My emotions and feelings changed dramatically throughout this incident. When the call was first received, I was anxious about what we would find on arrival. I was thinking about what actions we needed to take and trying to concentrate on arriving safely but as quickly as possible. When we arrived outside everything changed; the sounds we heard – screaming – what we saw – the door being only partially open. My senses went into overdrive (they still do on some calls).

At this point I was nervous but professionalism took over and I composed myself, preparing to take control. Once I walked through the door I realised I was faced with children and a very distraught wife. My feelings changed; how on earth I was going to manage this scene, take control of the wife and manage three young children? I remember thinking that the children should not be witnessing a resuscitation attempt or experiencing such distress in their young lives. Professionalism took over from my personal feelings of sadness, and I arranged for others to give support to the children and comfort the wife in another room. By this point, although not alone in the situation, I was feeling a large amount of responsibility to achieve a positive outcome for my patient. Unfortunately this did not happen, the patient died.

When the time came to end our efforts, my thoughts turned to breaking the news to the family. How was I going to do this, what was I going to say? In a professional but caring manner I told the family, my colleagues helped support me and the family, and this made things easier, but it was still very difficult and something I will never get used to doing.

It was after breaking the bad news and whilst clearing up that I felt guilty that we hadn't saved the children's dad, the wife's husband. Following the incident I felt confused about the cause of collapse and what support there would be (or not) for the children. How could they go back to school? Their lives would never be the same again.

After a while, a matter of days later, I finally felt contentment that we had done all we could do for everyone involved and there was nothing more we could have done to change the outcome of the situation. Reflecting now, I feel privileged to have been a part of that team, a part of that family's life for the short space of time and proud to call myself a paramedic and represent the profession.

As Box 12.1 begins to explore, individuals need to understand their reactions and emotions and reconcile these in relation to the situation encountered. An understanding of the potential personal consequences of some of the situations you may encounter is explored in the next section of this chapter.

How do you know if a situation has affected you?

Case studies are used to explain and explore how situations may affect the individual. Case Study 12.2 explains the normal feelings of a paramedic when responsibility for the patient is solely theirs.

CASE STUDY 12.2

When I started working as a paramedic I was worried about every patient I'd left at home, even when I had no doubt that they did not require hospital treatment at the time. I think this is quite a natural response and it eases with time. Certain jobs stay with me, not necessarily because they are typically traumatic, all for different reasons. The first death I saw stayed with me for quite some time, I had never experienced this prior to my paramedic career. I know when something is bothering me, that if I have any trouble getting to sleep followed by a work-related dream then it is clearly playing on my mind. Secondly, I'm a very conscientious person, if I need to go over something several times then that's a pretty good indicator that I've been affected.

Everyone is different and everyone will react to different situations. One piece of advice: if you internalise feelings then you will need to learn to share your feelings and concerns. One of the most helpful tools to have prior to beginning a career in paramedicine is a solid support network. This will expand through your career to include mentors, tutors and colleagues, as they will be the most likely to understand – being in similar situations.

As explained by the student paramedic's comments and reinforced by the comments in Case Study 12.2, sometimes the jobs that stay with you and concern you the most are not the ones you expect.

Case Study 12.2 describes normal responses but also recognises the value of going over something – reflecting on it. The responses described in Case Study 12.3 are more extreme and concerning.

⌀ Refer to Chapter 3 for more detail on reflection.

CASE STUDY 12.3

I had a concentrated three-week period where I had some very nasty jobs – there didn't seem to be any let-up at all. I thought I was fine until, on standby one night in the rapid response vehicle (RRV), I was reading a book with the interior light on and kept jumping out of my skin at the slightest thing. Everything from occasional traffic noise to the shadows of the trees on the windscreen had me jumping and jittering. I knew this wasn't right and it wasn't doing me any good. I dread to think what my vital signs were during this period. The best way I can explain it is that I felt as though I was in a constant state of high alert. I spoke to a friend (also a paramedic) about this, and he told me to Google 'exaggerated startle response/reflex'. This described what I was feeling exactly and I was shocked to read that 89% of people suffering early signs of post-traumatic stress disorder (PTSD) present in this way. I was able to take some time off from frontline duties and I returned to normal. The important point here is that I didn't realise I had been affected – I just knew something wasn't right.

The feeling that something is not right, described by the paramedic in Case Study 12.3, highlights the importance of understanding yourself. Had the paramedic been working on an ambulance, as part of a crew, instead of on a RRV it may have been that colleagues would have noticed this behaviour change too. The value of supportive networks should not be underestimated.

⌀ Refer to Chapter 13 for more detail on the subject of PTSD.

Remember, the case studies included are from registered clinicians and not from student paramedics. The responsibilities of clinicians are much greater than those of student paramedics. This is an important distinction to make, but it is also wise for you to read about the experiences of paramedics. It is good to be prepared with the knowledge that paramedics experience an array of emotions resulting from patient encounters, and sometimes need assistance/support to manage any adverse effects. The next chapter will consider further how you can build up your own resilience and access support as a paramedic.

Suggested reading

Whitnell, J. (2012) Abnormal psychology: an introduction. In A.Y. Blaber (ed.) *Foundations for Paramedic Practice: A Theoretical Perspective* (2nd edn). Maidenhead: Open University Press.

Search for books and articles on reflection and PTSD.

Read your university notes from lectures.

13 RESILIENCE AND SUPPORT

The career you have chosen is a stressful one. How can caring, on an almost daily basis, for people who are in pain, distressed, ill and sometimes dying not be stressful? As mentioned in previous chapters, understanding yourself is one of the most important aspects of keeping mentally and physically fit to do your job. The subject of resilience is addressed in paramedic studies, although it may be timetabled and discussed as 'managing and recognising stress in yourself and others', rather than as purely 'resilience'.

Reflection: points to consider

When you are in the clinical environment, what things do you find stressful?

Do you think that when you are a registered paramedic you will find the same things stressful as you do now, as a student?

Discuss stressors with your mentor and compare your results.

In Chapter 12 students and paramedics discussed a variety of situations they have found themselves in, all of which were stressful for various reasons. Gopee and Galloway (2009) identify sources of stress in health-care workers and have grouped them in the categories listed in Table 13.1.

Table 13.1 introduces some sources of stress that you may not have previously considered, such as restructuring and lack of job availability. What stresses you as a student is different from some of the considerations of registered health-care staff. Some areas remain a consistent source of stress for students and staff alike, such as shift work. Obviously as your role changes and evolves the sources of stress will also change, but the one thing that probably will not is the fact that you will experience some form of stress.

Table 13.1 Sources of stress categorised into groups (Gopee and Galloway 2009)

Work–life imbalance	Working with temporary staff
Lack of availability of resources	Competing demands for time
Paperwork and bureaucracy	Staffing challenges such as sickness and vacancies
Professional relationships	Lack of teamwork
Cliques	Inefficient systems of work
Clinical incidents	Shift work
Off-duty/rota	Changes
Redeployment	Restructuring
Lack of job security	Lack of job availability
Financial constraints	

Reflection: points to consider

List the physical changes that you experience when you are stressed.

Recognising symptoms of stress

If you do not learn to recognise manifestations of stress in yourself you are less likely to tune into any of your colleagues or patients or families of patients exhibiting stressed behaviour. As a paramedic you are part of a wider team of people, even if you work as a solo responder or as part of a two-person crew. You and your paramedic family are there to help each other, and you will not be able to do that if you cannot recognise stress in yourself.

Definition: Stress

Hawkins and Shohet (2012) define stress as 'a state of fatigue, ill-health and at times depression caused by distressing, strenuous and emotionally overwhelming situations'.

Hawkins and Shohet (2012) and Gopee and Galloway (2009) discuss the physical and behavioural manifestations of experiencing stress. Box 13.1 contains a list of the various symptoms of stress. This list is not exhaustive, and I am sure you can add more physical changes of your own from the list you created for the reflection point on the previous page.

Box 13.1 A list of the symptoms of stress

Overtiredness

Loss of appetite

Insomnia

Headaches/migraine

Diarrhoea/indigestion

Inability to concentrate

Paranoid thoughts

Avoiding friends/colleagues

Increased alcohol intake, overeating

Sudden mood swings

Short-term and transient stress is not a negative experience. Think about any interview or examination: feeling a little stressed raises your adrenaline, heightens your awareness and reactions, and makes you ready for action. Too much and periods of prolonged stress are when the problems begin.

It is true that in certain situations others recognise there is a problem before we do, as the examples provided in Box 13.2 help to illustrate. For this reason, colleagues working together are in a unique position to identify any changes in each other's behaviour, personality or ability to work. This is an important informal strategy, but one that can be effective in enabling the individual to assess, evaluate any issues and act to improve their physical and mental well-being.

In Case Study 12.2, the paramedic referred to the term 'post-traumatic stress disorder', and this will be explained briefly below.

Box 13.2 How can recognising stress in your colleagues help them?

:📢: **Paramedic response:** I had a major row with my crewmate when I thought she was exhibiting symptoms of stress. After a few days she apologised and admitted a specific job had touched a nerve and she needed to talk to someone about her feelings. Eventually, I was glad I had had the courage to mention my concerns to her.

:📢: **Paramedic/PEd response:** I worked with a colleague who after a series of serious jobs where patients died seemed to shy away from the action. We had worked together for a while, and this was unusual for him. I found time to discuss this and found that he was finding cardiac arrests hard to manage and experiencing other physical symptoms. He accessed help and after a few months the situation improved, but if he had not been encouraged to talk and get help early on, things may have got worse. He needed me to bring this to his attention and stop him denying there was a problem.

Post-traumatic stress disorder

PTSD is an anxiety disorder, first noted in war veterans. Stress is the cause of PTSD and can be seen in victims of trauma or observers who witness or are involved in the event, hence it is of particular significance to paramedics and those working in the emergency services (Whitnell 2012). PTSD is also linked with a high suicide rate. The common signs and symptoms are presented in Box 13.3.

Box 13.3 Signs and symptoms/presentation of individuals with PTSD (Whitnell 2012: 105)

PTSD occurs, in equal number, in people who are victims of trauma, in observers who witness trauma or in those who are actually involved in the event as workers (e.g. blue-light services).

PTSD can occur in children following a traumatic event for them, such as the divorce of their parents.

PTSD sufferers have a high suicide rate.

The paradoxical symptoms of PTSD encompass the following:

- Anxiety, caused by the fear of the past experience. In this situation the person will try to avoid anything associated with the trauma.
- The person may lose their memory of the event. They may experience intrusive and unwanted thoughts, such as flashbacks and nightmares.
- The person describes themselves as being psychologically numb or emotionally shut down. In this situation they are unable to find pleasure in things and cannot look to the future.
- Conversely, the person may have symptoms of hyper-arousal. This describes a state where the person startles easily, cannot sleep or concentrate. They may also be irritable and easily angered.

Long-term exposure to consistent stress, with low resilience, can predispose the individual to a state of exhaustion (burnout), as explained below.

Burnout

Burnout is the term used when a person suffers long-term, consistent stress and is unable to manage or cope with the cause of stress in an effective way. The value of recognising symptoms of stress, and taking action to combat them, is that it may help to prevent burnout. This could equally apply to you or your colleagues; you need to look after yourself and each other, in order that you can look after others.

The following definition also describes some of the indicators of burnout:

Definition: Burnout

Burnout is 'a state of emotional and physical exhaustion accompanied by a lack of interest in one's job, low trust in others, a loss of caring, cynicism towards others, self-deprecation, low morale and a deep sense of failure' (Hawkins and Shohet 2012).

Individual responses to stress are as unique as the individual themselves. Some people are naturally more resilient than others, but before further discussion definitions of resilience require consideration.

What is resilience?

Definition: Resilience

Resilience is 'an ability to rebound from adversity and overcome difficult circumstances in one's life' (Marsh 1996: 543) or 'a process of adaptation to adversity' (Newman 2003: 42).

Throughout our lives, we encounter difficult experiences. If your chosen career places you in situations that are difficult, variously stressful or outside the realms of those usually experienced by lay people, the need to develop good, positive coping mechanisms is strong. The above definitions are not specific to paramedic practice, but Box 13.4 may help you to appreciate how important resilience is to paramedics.

Box 13.4 Define what resilience means to you?

📖 **Student paramedic response:** Resilience is the ability to bounce back from adversity. If you've made it this far and gained a place on a paramedic programme you've certainly already got a measure of resilience!

I think resilience is made up of a number of factors including your social support, outlook on life and sense of humour. All of these can affect whether you approach difficulties in a positive way. I think resilience can be developed to deal with the unique aspects of paramedic work, but it comes from the foundation of the type of person you are – if you have more of an 'Eeyore' personality then becoming a paramedic is probably not for you.

🚨 **Paramedic response:** Resilience is the ability to protect yourself against the extreme stresses, pressures and sights we see in our profession and the ability to have strategies and plans in place to manage and cope with this accordingly.

Paramedic mentor/PEd response: To me resilience can be seen as a kind of toughness, the capacity to recover quickly from difficulties. This should not be confused with hardness and a lack of compassion – quite the opposite. Studies into burnout have shown that this is more likely to present as a lack of caring than being over-emotional.

Academic response: Resilience is your ability to absorb, manage, cope with, organise and come to terms with anything that is personally difficult for you, without it having detrimental effects on your physical and mental well-being.

Academic response: Many studies show that resilience training/ education is something that needs to be included in the paramedic curriculum. We need to prepare our students as best we can for the role they are about to undertake. The difficult part is to figure out just how we can teach resilience. So many variables are involved: personality type, support networks, coping mechanisms, locus of control and distracting behaviour.

The various comments in Box 13.4 recognise some commonality in the way resilience is thought of and present a variety of examples for you to consider in the following reflection exercise.

Reflection: points to consider

Think about all of the definitions of resilience. Which one makes most sense to you?

As mentioned by the contributors, individual personality characteristics have a part to play in the presence or development of resilience.

Characteristics of resilient individuals

Denz-Penhey and Murdoch (2008) examined the characteristics of people who were resilient. They discovered that there seemed to be five areas that were of importance in the individuals' lives (see Table 13.2). They state that the characteristics and dimensions of the self listed in Table 13.2 enable resilient individuals to develop a suite of coping skills that support them through challenging times.

Table 13.2 The five dimensions of resilience in adults' lives (Denz-Penhey and Murdoch (2008)

Connectedness to social environment
Connectedness to family
Connectedness to the physical environment
Connectedness to a sense of inner wisdom (experiential spirituality)
Personal psychology with a supportive mind-set and a way of living that supports the individual's values

Connectedness to family is of obvious interest to those of us supporting student paramedics. If connectedness to family is helpful in developing resilience, then we can appreciate there is an added stressor for student paramedics who are living away from home and managing difficult situations without their established support networks.

𝒞 Refer to Chapter 2 and the comments from students on support networks.

Can resilience be developed?

There is growing evidence that resilience can be learned. Sometimes cognitive behavioural therapy (CBT) may be useful. Investigate further if it is of interest to you.

Jackson et al. (2007) consider that resilience can be specifically strengthened and developed by individuals. Some of their suggestions are given in Box 13.5. Some of these are common sense and have been mentioned throughout this text as being natural processes and not something requiring specific effort.

Box 13.5 Suggestions to help develop resilience

Building positive professional relationships through networks and mentoring

Maintaining positivity through laughter, optimism and positive emotions

Developing emotional insight to understand your own risk and protective factors

Using life balance and spirituality to give your life meaning and coherence

Becoming more reflective to help you find emotional strength and obtain meaning from experiences

However, developing self-awareness is so important to your role as a student and as a registered paramedic. Be honest about each of the suggestions in Box 13.5 and seriously consider if any of the suggestions would help you learn more about yourself.

Reflection: points to consider

Refer back to the list of things that make you feel stressed you were asked to consider early in this chapter.

Reflect on how you manage these situations.

In light of the suggestions and strategies discussed in this chapter, do you now feel that you could do anything differently?

No matter how self-aware you are or how much resilience you possess or work on developing, you are likely to encounter, at some point, a situation or series of events that you feel inadequately prepared for or unable to cope with. It is important to have a plan for how to manage such events.

Who can you talk to?

As a student paramedic you have a host of services and facilities available to you, but you may not realise it, especially if you have not needed them before.

Formal

Students will have the raft of services of the university available to them. Although called by different names in different universities, there will be a formal structure of services and facilities available to students. Ask your lecturers or personal tutor for details, or check the web pages or visit the department yourself.

As a student paramedic you will have met staff from the occupational health department who manage health-care students' own health needs. For example, all health-care students will require immunisations and booster injections for specific diseases prior to exposure to patients. If a student is off sick after breaking their leg, for instance, the occupational health department will need to assess and confirm that the student is fit to go back to both academic study and the practice environment. This service may also be able to offer support that is specific to your needs, and is often an under-utilised resource.

If you are spending part of your studies working for an ambulance trust, you should be entitled to access the same services as employees, such as counselling and occupational health. You may also be able to access clinical supervision as a member of the ambulance trust, if these groups are available in your locality.

Non-formal

If you feel you just need an informal social network, there may be reflection groups that run in your faculty, among health-care students or specifically student paramedic groups. There is also value in peer learning or peer review, where student paramedics from varying cohorts meet informally and discuss their experiences, reflect on situations confidentially, and try to make sense of what has occurred in the practice environment. These may be student-led or facilitated by a member of academic or practice staff. However, this may not be a support system available in every institution.

Also consider professional forums or special interest groups. These may be open to students via the ambulance trust or within the university. This may enable you to enhance your learning in a certain area and improve your confidence, reducing stress that may occur when caring for certain patient groups, such as newborn babies. If you take control, by learning more and potentially becoming a specialist in a specific area, or particular patient group, it becomes less intimidating, less stressful and less likely to be the cause of any long-term stress.

What if it all becomes too much?

As we have said, it is wise to talk to someone. Read the comments below and the advice from academics and practitioners – these will provide you with some good tips and give you the confidence to know that you will not be the first student paramedic to find it tough, nor will you be the last.

Student paramedic comment: I think we all had a wobble or two whilst on the programme, wondering if we were cut out for paramedic work. It is something you go through on occasions. If you find things are getting on top of you then talk to someone you trust. Talk to your programme leader, lecturers or mentor, as they probably understand more of what you're facing than anyone else. It might not be something which signals that you shouldn't be a paramedic, it might just be that you need some extra support to get over a particular hurdle. Don't keep quiet and hope for the best – you can't care for others if you don't take care of yourself.

Box 13.6 What advice would you give to students who are really struggling and suffering?

Academic response: Get help. No programme of study or career is ever worth a disturbing personal sacrifice of being mentally and/ or physically ill. It is a fact that being a paramedic is not for everyone. You are not a failure. You can use all of your experiences and knowledge in another area perhaps. Talk to your lecturers; it may be that you can step off your programme with an academic qualification that you can take forward to another university course if you so wish. For example, successful completion of level 4 study will in most institutions enable you to leave with a certificate in higher education, or similar title. Your lecturers will not want to see you leave, but recognise that for some students this is the only option. They do not want you to be unhappy or unwell.

🎓 **Academic response:** Talk to whoever you feel most comfortable discussing your concerns with. This may be a colleague, mentor, loved one or member of academic staff. It doesn't really matter who you talk to, as long as you talk.

The answers to the question posed in Box 13.6 relate to advice that may be useful when considering if your career choice is right for you. The following reflection point is intended to help you better understand yourself as a student paramedic and a professional.

Reflection: points to consider

Some questions for you to consider and answer:

Your identity
What do I believe in?

What are my aspirations?

What will I stand up for?

Your coping capacity and development of your strengths
What do I need to know about what it takes to succeed out there?

What will I encounter for which I need to be prepared?

How can I develop critical thinking, creative thinking and a sense of humour to help me cope?

Feeling like you need help at some points during your studies is not a failing – indeed, it reminds you that you are human and you care about what you are trying to achieve. Academic and practice staff would rather have numerous students who find parts of their programme and life in practice hard than students who are oblivious to the needs of themselves, their colleagues and their patients. Caring for others is not an easy role and not one that it is easy to detach from once you have finished a shift – this is normal and something that as caring professionals we too have found our own way of coping with. There is help available and you are likely find a solution to suit you. Very often what is right for one student is not right for another – try whatever you think may help you!

Suggested reading

Denz-Penhey, H. and Murdoch, C. (2008) Personal resiliency: serious diagnosis and prognosis with unexpected quality outcomes. *Qualitative Health Research*, 18(3): 391–404.

Gopee, N. and Galloway, J. (2009) *Leadership and Management in Healthcare*. London: Sage.

Hawkins, P. and Shohet, R. (2012) *Supervision in the Helping Professions* (4th edn). Maidenhead: Open University Press.

Jackson, D., Firtko, A. and Edenborough, M. (2007) Personal resilience as a strategy for surviving and thriving in the face of workplace adversity: a literature review. *Journal of Advanced Nursing*, 60(1): 1–9.

Malkin, K.F. (1994) A standard for professional development: the use of self and peer review; learning contracts and reflection in clinical practice. *Journal of Nursing Management*, 2: 143–148.

Marsh, D.T. (1996) Marilyn ... and other offspring. *Journal of the California Alliance for the Mentally Ill*, 27(3): 543–562.

McAllister, M. and McKinnon, J. (2008) The importance of teaching and learning resilience in the health disciplines: A critical review of the literature. *Nurse Education Today*, October.

Newman, R. (2003) Providing direction on the road to resilience. *Behavioural Health Management*, 23(4): 42–43.

NHS Employers (2006) *Model Bullying and Harassment Policy*. London: NHS Employers. Available at: http://www.nhsemployers.org/toolkit/search.cfm (accessed 18 January 2015).

Randle, J., Stevenson, K. and Grayling, I. (2007) Reducing workplace bullying in healthcare organisations. *Nursing Standard*, 21(22): 49–56.

Whitnell, J. (2012) Abnormal psychology: an introduction. In A.Y. Blaber (ed.) *Foundations for Paramedic Practice: A Theoretical Perspective* (2nd edn). Maidenhead: Open University Press.

14 FITTING IN

One of the most challenging aspects of starting a new job is the element of fitting in. The student paramedic experiences this because of the number of transitions they go through during and after their studies. The student feels pressure to fit into their cohort or group at university and then, usually reported as being more of a challenge, also attempt to fit into the clinical environment.

Top tips from students about fitting in

Student paramedics are continually learning about the culture of the staff within the ambulance service and the wider organisation, the NHS ambulance trust, where they undertake the practice element of their programme. Generally it presents a challenge because it is such a different environment from that which students have previously experienced.

> **Student paramedic comment:** It always takes a couple of shifts before you begin to feel you're fitting in. I found offering to make tea whenever the opportunity arose worked wonders. Cake is the currency of acceptance in the ambulance service: buy it, make it, but above all bring it into the station and dish it out – you'll make friends for life.

> **Student paramedic comment:** It's common sense really; show some willingness to do the tasks you don't have to (like washing up in the crew room) and word gets round that you're 'OK'. Check the kit bags are all complete on the truck (apart from helping the crew, you get to know where everything is if you suddenly need a particular bag when on a job), be the one who disinfects the trolley, remakes the linen and prepares the truck for the next job – it all works in your favour.

As the two students' comments above and the comments from the paramedic in Box 14.1 make clear, being enthusiastic whilst also being prepared to do more mundane tasks seems to be a way to earn your initial acceptance.

Box 14.1 Any advice you would pass on to students about fitting in at their local ambulance station or with a crew?

Paramedic response: Most staff will arrive 15 minutes before their shift start time; this is to check over the ambulance and equipment and to prevent their colleagues being called out for a late job. It's a good idea to do your best to arrive early so they don't have to wait for you. Making tea usually goes down well – if you really want to push the boat out, turn up with cakes or biscuits! Be outgoing, ask questions and be a team player. You are likely to go to various ambulance stations, it can be overwhelming – try to introduce yourself each time you meet someone new. It will go down well and you will get a good reputation for being friendly.

Paramedic mentor/PEd response: The organisational culture of the ambulance service can be a strange animal. Humour, particularly of the dark kind, is common and this can often be a bit of a culture shock to students. Don't judge your colleagues for this. Dark humour is a bona-fide coping mechanism and is common amongst emergency services personnel. Be friendly and open with people, willing to listen and learn. Don't go in with the attitude that you know more because of your academic studies. Many excellent ambulance staff who do not have academic qualifications or have not reached paramedic level have a wealth of practical experience to share.

The mentor/PEd response in Box 14.1 refers to organisational culture and the uniqueness of ambulance service culture. This is explored in a little more detail in the next section of this chapter.

Organisational culture

The ambulance service has a military background, and this is well documented (Craggs and Blaber 2008; Newton 2012a, 2012b; Richardson 1974). As a consequence of these military roots, with a hierarchical structure and clear chains of command, it is not surprising that the ambulance service developed along similar lines. This may be one of the reasons why students and newly registered paramedics get very used to making the tea and cleaning up. The concept of organisational culture is one that is difficult to define, with academics disagreeing on definitions (Blaber and Harris 2014). The definition below suits the requirements of this text perfectly and is something that every reader will clearly understand.

Definition: Organisational culture

'The way we do things around here' (Balogun and Hailey 2008).

On occasions, the way things have been done has stayed the same for many years. Practices and cultural norms may be initially shocking for the student paramedic – an example of this being the humour used by staff.

It must be remembered that the paramedic profession is undergoing professionalisation, and practices/cultural norms of a few years ago are no longer as acceptable. The vast majority of paramedics have welcomed the professionalisation and act as consummate professionals all of the time. It is possible that student paramedics may meet a few trust employees who do not adhere to the same professional standards as paramedics. The student paramedic needs to be able to distinguish the differences, with the help of their mentor/PEd. In Box 14.2, contributors provide some of their own advice.

Box 14.2 What advice would you give to students about the culture of the ambulance services?

Paramedic mentor/PEd response: Whilst it is initially alien to students, most will find their colleagues becoming like extended family. The experiences you have with colleagues and the amount of time you spend together will develop into a special bond the strength of which cannot be underestimated.

Academic response: The organisational culture of the ambulance service can initially seem daunting. Many people have known each other for years. The higher education route into paramedic practice is still a relatively new one and is taking some getting used to by some people. This will change over time, and it is of use to remember that you are an advertisement for this system.

Give yourself time to observe, listen to and appreciate the ambulance service culture. As the responses in Box 14.2 highlight, it will take to time to understand the close community that is the ambulance service.

Suggested reading

Balogun, J. and Hailey, V.H. (2008) *Exploring Strategic Change* (3rd edn). London: Financial Times/Prentice Hall.

Blaber, A.Y. and Harris, G. (eds) (2014) *Clinical Leadership for Paramedics*. Maidenhead: Open University Press.

Craggs, B. and Blaber, A.Y. (2008) Consideration of history. In A.Y. Blaber (ed.) *Foundations for Paramedic Practice: A Theoretical Perspective*. Maidenhead: Open University Press.

Newton, A. and Hodge, D. (2012a) The ambulance service: the past, present and future. *Journal of Paramedic Practice*, 4(5): 303–305.

Newton, A. (2012b) The ambulance service: the past, present and future. *Journal of Paramedic Practice*, 4(6): 365–366.

Orr, J.S. (1989) *The Organizational Culture Perspective*. Pacific Grove, CA: Brooks/Cole.

Richardson, R. (1974) *Larrey: Surgeon to Napoleon's Imperial Guard*. London: John Murray.

Savage, J. (2000) The culture of 'culture' in National Health Service policy implementation. *Nursing Inquiry*, 7: 230–238.

PART 4
Transition to registration

15 ARE YOU READY?

This chapter explores the thoughts and feelings of students and paramedics as they come to the end of their period of study. It is easy at this point to feel totally comfortable in your role as a student paramedic: you know exactly what is expected of you, you and your mentor/PEd form a team and know most people in your base station/area. Any change to this status quo may make you a little fearful, in addition to the thought that you will soon be completing your studies and need to get a job as a registered paramedic. One thing that is quite common is that students in the final year of their studies experience a temporary reduction in their confidence levels.

Confidence

For some students the loss of confidence does not happen, for others it is associated with their academic work. For the vast majority, it is linked to the clinical area and their performance in practice. It happens to different students at different points, but if you expect it you can try and manage it, to stop fear and worry getting the better of you. The wise words of a programme leader are retold in the student's comment below.

> **Student paramedic comment:** The words of my programme leader will stay with me for ever. One day we were having a few wobbles about finishing our studies, and this is what he said:
>
> > In the first year, you were incompetent but you didn't know it! You were just enjoying flying around in the ambulance on blue lights thinking how fun it all was. Later you were still incompetent but were beginning to realise it, understanding that you needed to learn a lot. Now you have reached the stage where you are competent but you don't yet realise it. You know lots of stuff and you can do this job but you lack the full confidence

you need. The final stage of the process (stage four) is when you are competent and you realise it. You *can* do this job, and though there will always be new things to learn you will have confidence to meet the demands of the day.

He told us that we were exactly where he expected us to be at that time and that he had every confidence in us. He also said it probably wouldn't be until we had graduated and been registered paramedics for a few months before we would feel we had reached 'stage four'. His chat with us really made a difference. I'll never forget it.

The student nearing the end of their studies will be wiser than they were at the beginning, more aware of their professional responsibilities and, of course, that is scary but it signals that you are taking your role seriously and understand what is expected of you, unlike you ever did in year 1 of your studies. Having made it to the final year of your studies is a cause for celebration. The reality check of soon being a registered paramedic will probably play on your mind a little; this will be different for all of your fellow students. If you experience a drop in confidence, see Box 15.1 for some advice that may help.

Box 15.1 What advice would you give to help students increase their confidence?

Academic response: Gaining your paramedic registration is like passing your driving test. You have met the minimum standard and will really start to learn to drive after you have received your test certificate. Don't expect to know everything just because you have gained your registration, and try not to be too hard on yourself. Confidence will develop. You would not be where you are now if you didn't have what it takes!

As explained in Box 15.1, you need to have realistic expectations of your-self – you are not going to know it all or have an in-depth knowledge about every illness, injury and patient condition that you encounter. But what you do have are *the tools* to continue learning, researching, developing, reflecting and improving yourself as a registered paramedic. Do not forget or negate the wider lessons you learnt whilst in higher education – they will be useful.

 🖉 Refer to Chapter 3 for more on reflection.

Ideas on how to prepare yourself in the last year of study/practice

Having explored the potential loss of confidence, it is wise to investigate the thoughts of contributors about how best to prepare for your final year of studies and the time in practice leading up to registration. The following comment is of course personal to one student, but contains several wider points about study and practice.

Student paramedic comment: In your final year on placement you really need to step up and push yourself forward to do things. I found at times I was 'hiding behind the paperwork' (at each job someone fills out a form detailing patient condition, observations, interventions, etc.). I realised that I had got into the habit of grabbing the clipboard and starting to write at most jobs, but this meant I wasn't getting to perform procedures. This may be fine in year 1 and the start of year 2, but you need to make sure you're increasingly getting exposure to practice too. I mentioned it to my mentor and we agreed that I would do most of the attending at jobs from then on.

At my other station my mentor there told me that in the last year he would just carry my bags and I would attend everything so that I got used to 'being in the hot seat' whilst he was still there to support me. This was great as I developed a lot of confidence and honed my skills.

I found myself reading loads on clinical skills during my third year – stuff we had been taught in years 1 and 2 that I wanted to keep refreshing myself on. You can get engrossed in writing your dissertation during year 3 (if you are on a BSc programme) to the detriment of keeping up to date on your skills knowledge. It's about finding a balance.

You have to put together a portfolio of work showing continual professional development – which you add to throughout your career as a requirement to keep your registration. It's probably best to start this at the end of year 1 and into year 2 of your programme, rather than leave it until the last few months of year 3 (or 2 depending on the length of your studies) as you need to put loads of stuff in it to show prospective employers. The sort of things they want to see are: reflective essays on jobs you've been to, courses you may have attended as part of uni or in addition to uni, things you've done in support of your profession, etc.

Previous students told us that they took their portfolios to interviews and the interviewers never looked at them. At my interview they made a point of looking through it, so you never can tell!

The student comments above indicate that the juggling act mentioned in Chapters 2 and 3 continues to the end of your studies. It is wise to reflect on how you are working in the practice environment with your mentors/PEds. As the student above mentions, a note-taking routine had been established with his mentor that would not have equipped the student well once the responsibility for patient care was his alone. The balance between revising clinical skills and theoretical work is something you have been working on from early on in your studies – it is probably more daunting now as the importance of knowing it all becomes more significant, as the advice given in Box 15.2 recognises.

Box 15.2 Advice about your final year of study

🎓 **Academic advice:** Many students go into panic mode in the final year of study. This is completely normal, especially with the pressure of assignments and clinical examinations to face. Remember – you are nearly there. Pull out all the stops for the final push towards registration and ask for support when you feel you need it, even if it takes the form of a good moan over a cup of coffee!

🚨 **Paramedic mentor/PEd advice:** If you have a good mentor he/she will be letting you take the lead without your really knowing it. You will lead jobs, making all decisions and carrying out all interventions, with your mentor only as a 'psychological safety blanket'.

As alluded to in Box 15.2 and in the student's comments, your mentor/PEd will probably have been letting you take the lead for much of your final year and usually you will have been doing well. It seems to be when you start to think about registration that doubt creeps in and confidence dips a little. Your mentor/PEd should be able to help you with this, provided you let them know how you are feeling. Also remember that you should have a period of preceptorship to complete once you start your first role as a paramedic. This will be discussed in Chapter 17.

⤻ Refer to Chapter 2 for more on support networks.

Of course, you will need to apply for registration to the HCPC, and the next section gives some guidance about this.

Applying for registration

Take advice from your programme team about the best time to apply for registration. Usually the university will send a pass list to the HCPC and your registration form will then be cross-checked with the pass list. Your registration will usually be processed within 3–6 weeks. The HCPC cannot process your application without the pass list from the university stating you have satisfied all of the criteria to become a registered paramedic, so it is probably best not to send your application form in too early, as the academic in Box 15.3 also explains.

Box 15.3 When is the best time to apply for registration?

🎓 **Academic response:** Most programme staff will advise you about the date when your results and placement hours have been ratified at the academic board. Ask the programme team for advice on the HCPC process, but it is usually quite simple, involving the completion of a form (available from the HCPC website), verification of photographs, identification and qualifications.

Portfolio development

As the student comment earlier in the chapter mentions, you may also leave your university with a portfolio. Some programmes will have the portfolio as a credited module/unit, for other programmes it will be an additional piece of work that you should complete before attending ambulance trusts for interview. Some students say interview panels examine their portfolio, others may not be asked, but taking your portfolio with you to any interview is now widely expected (see Box 15.4).

Box 15.4 Do you need your portfolio for interviews?

🎓 **Academic response:** It is always good practice to take your portfolio with you to any interview you may attend. This is something you will continue with throughout your career and is a condition of your HCPC registration, so it is a good idea to start this early. A good CPD portfolio will go a long way to showing a student's competence and enthusiasm. It can be the one thing that makes you stand out from the crowd at interview.

The reason why portfolios are introduced at undergraduate level is that the content of a portfolio will help form part of the continuing professional development (CPD) record that you are required to keep and maintain as a registered paramedic.

Continuing professional development

It is wise to look at the HCPC definition of CPD, as this may differ from other generic definitions or those for other professions.

Definition: Continuing professional development

CPD is 'a range of learning activities through which health professionals maintain and develop throughout their career to ensure that they retain their capacity to practise safely, effectively and legally within their evolving scope of practice' (HCPC 2014: 1).

As can be seen from the above definition, CPD is closely linked to maintaining your registration as a paramedic. The HCPC (2014: 12) lists five requirements of registrants in respect of CPD (see Table 15.1).

Table 15.1 HCPC standards for CPD

Registrants must:
1. maintain a continuous, up-to-date and accurate record of their CPD activities;
2. demonstrate that their CPD activities are a mixture of learning activities relevant to current or future practice;
3. seek to ensure that their CPD has contributed to the quality of their practice and service delivery;
4. seek to ensure that their CPD benefits the service user;
5. upon request, present a written profile (which must be their own work and supported by evidence) explaining how they have met the standards for CPD.

Table 15.1 refers to a written profile; you may also hear this being referred to by clinicians as a portfolio. The HCPC guidance is generic to all registrants of the HCPC, it is not specific to paramedics, so you are not being asked to do anything more than other HCPC-registered health-care professionals. There is no shortage of guidance, should you require it. For instance, the HCPC provides a list of guidance and examples of types of CPD activity (Harris and Fellows 2012).

The HCPC randomly chooses paramedics to be audited each year. These chosen profiles are assessed by a CPD team, one of whom will be a paramedic. There are three possible outcomes of this assessment:

(a)   you meet the standards;
(b)   more information is needed; or
(c)   your profile does not meet the standards (you may be offered 3 months to meet the standards or recommendation will be made that your registration should end).

A registrant has 2 years after registration before the HCPC can ask to see their profile. This time should be spent developing your profile along the guidelines provided by the HCPC and not necessarily in the format you have previously been using.

Participation in CPD events and reflecting on their value to you and your service users is important in order to maintain your registration. The College of Paramedics works on your behalf to provide a suite of CPD activities, as mentioned in Box 15.5. These are available to both members of the College of Paramedics and non-members, but there is a cost difference. In addition to the College of Paramedics CPD events, many universities now have student paramedic forums and active student groups which host national study days, so keep alert for these events too.

Box 15.5 What kind of CPD events did you find it useful to take part in during your first year of registration?

🚨 **Paramedic mentor/PEd response:** The College of Paramedics holds many informative CPD days across the UK. This is great for keeping you up to date with current practice and highlighting any changes that will arise in the future. It also shows that you have taken the trouble to attend, that you have been bothered enough.

The requirements on you both as a student and registrant are commensurate with those of a professional, and maintaining your registration is of course a prime way for you to show you are working at the correct standard. Whilst discussion has moved from final-year study to the requirements for gaining and maintaining registration in this chapter, it is important to discuss securing your first employed position as a paramedic. Chapter 16 will continue to offer guidance towards employment.

Suggested reading

Harris, G. and Fellows, R. (2012) Continuing professional development: pre and post registration. In A.Y. Blaber (ed.) *Foundations for Paramedic Practice: A Theoretical Perspective*. Maidenhead: Open University Press.

Health and Care Professions Council (2011) *How to Fill in your Registration Renewal Form*. London: HCPC. Available at: http://www.hpc-uk.org/assets/documents/10002C21100009C0Renewal_form_how_to_guide.pdf

Health and Care Professions Council (2014) *Continuing Professional Development and Your Registration*. London: HCPC. Available at: http://www.hcpc-uk.org.uk/assets/documents/10001314CPD_and_your_registration.pdf (accessed 18 January 2015).

16 GETTING YOUR FIRST JOB

As has been alluded to throughout the text, the student will experience a series of transitions. One of these is the significant transition from the role of student to the role of employee. Usually the student is applying for jobs before they have completed their studies, as the process of becoming employed as a paramedic may take several months.

What ambulance service do you want to work for?

In some respects this decision is similar to the one you made when you decided on your university choices. Assuming that your NHS ambulance trust is employing newly registered paramedics, you will have the choice of applying to the trust where you have been working as a student paramedic or applying to another trust in a different location. The responses in Box 16.1 from the student paramedic and paramedic explain that their decision-making was personal to them, just as it will be for you.

∂ Refer to Chapter 2 for more on support networks and Chapter 13 for more on resilience.

> **Box 16.1 What things do you consider when applying for your first paramedic role?**
>
> 📖 **Student paramedic response:** The great thing about being a paramedic is that there are opportunities all over the country, and overseas once you have a few years' experience. I wanted to stay in the area I was educated, not just because I live there but when comparing ambulance trusts I felt that the trust in my area offered more opportunity for development and allowed their paramedics to carry out procedures which other trusts didn't (like intubation). Having learnt these skills, I didn't want to lose them.

Paramedic response: When I applied for my first job I discussed my options in depth with my family, close friends, course-mates and tutors. I applied for two trusts, the one where I had been educated and one where I grew up and where my family live. When I was offered both jobs I was faced with a tough decision. One of my tutors advised me to stay within the trust I knew, as she felt this would be easier for my transition to paramedic. I did not take her advice! I went to an unfamiliar trust; my primary reason for this was to be closer to my family. I also wanted to be accepted as a paramedic, not an ex-student, when beginning my first job. The post I was offered in the trust I knew was at the station I'd been on placement at from day 1 as a student. I felt I might still be viewed as a student. This may suit other students. In hindsight I will never know if I made the best decision. I know I made a good decision and the right one for me. I have been really well supported as a newly qualified paramedic. I was fortunate to have an excellent mentor/preceptor and staff have been very welcoming. But I can see the benefits of staying within the service where you have been a student. Familiarising yourself with a new service is stressful at what can be an overwhelming time.

Paramedic mentor/PEd response: Many students choose to apply to the trust they have undertaken placement with, as this will have become familiar to them and 'the road they know' over their programme of study. This really is an individual decision and will differ from person to person.

Academic response: There are a few things to take into consideration when deciding where to work. Are you happy to relocate or do you want to stay near to home and support networks? All ambulance trusts vary in what they have to offer. Would you like to specialise in the future, and how? It may be that different trusts offer different opportunities and it may be worth taking this into account when you are considering this in years to come.

As the paramedic mentor/PEd response in Box 16.1 explains, some students choose to stay within the trust they know and have worked within as a student. But you may not be working in the same station you have been in previously. For some people this is a positive, for others a negative. Some students want to relocate and start with a new ambulance trust in a registered paramedic capacity, as they worry about being still known as 'the student', as alluded to in the comments above. You will need to weigh this up and make the decision for yourself.

Once you have decided on your employment choices, you will need to apply for a paramedic job.

Job application

Apart from your university interview, this may be the first job interview you have attended. Most job vacancies and applications are managed by the NHS jobs website. It is usual practice that ambulance trusts come and speak to students who are about to qualify. This usually involves a presentation and question-and-answer session. The NHS ambulance trusts will be selling themselves to you, in the same way that the universities do at open days. You will usually be supported by your university at this point, and guidance will be given to you about the job application process.

Advice on preparing your supporting statement

As the student paramedic response in Box 16.2 indicates, the job application process may coincide with final assessments of your programme. For this reason, it is easy to feel pressured and not apply yourself as much as is needed to one or other, but you should keep your eyes on your goal of becoming employed as a paramedic and work at both.

Along with your personal details, employment history and qualifications, most application forms for any role in the NHS also ask you to provide a supporting statement. This is your chance to sell yourself on paper. Just as your university lecturers only had your UCAS personal statement to read before shortlisting you for interview, the same applies to the supporting statement part of your application form. A paramedic job description will be available to you, along with the forms. This is really important. You need to reflect the aspects of the job description when you are writing your personal statement. Additionally, the reader needs to get a sense of who you are. Table 16.1 provides some advice about preparing your supporting statement.

Table 16.1 Advice on preparing a supporting statement

Be methodical:
- Is where you started different from where you are now?
- What have you learnt?
- Skills, personal attributes, knowledge

Be professional

Make sure there are no mistakes

Tell the reader what you want them to know

Have an idea of what the reader wants to hear

Read and highlight the main points of the job description

If there is a list of desirable and essential attributes, use them and ensure you address them in your supporting statement

Use your module/unit content (learning outcomes in your handbooks) to assist your structure

Think about joining relevant associations, professional or voluntary groups, committees, research interest groups, etc.

Once you have considered the points addressed in Table 16.1, you will be ready to start writing. Do not underestimate how long it will take you to construct, amend, rewrite and recheck a supporting statement. It is not something that can be rushed, as your future employment may depend upon it.

Once you have written your first draft:

- Read it through again.
- Ask a member of the teaching team also to read and make comment.
- Be critical.
- Does it:
  - have no mistakes?
  - have a professional focus?
  - have a logical progression?
  - accurately represent what you know and who you are?
  - represent your strengths?

Once you have a second or third draft of your supporting statement it may be ready to send. There will usually be a gap between the closing date for applications and interview dates, during which time you can refocus on your studies. Remember, any job offer will be conditional on you success-fully completing your programme of paramedic study.

The following section provides some advice in order to prepare for interview.

Advice prior to interview

There are some practical things that you can do to prepare prior to your interview. These are presented in Table 16.2.

Table 16.2 Practical things you can do prior to interview

Review your supporting statement critically. Remind yourself what was written in it.
Devise some questions you think an interviewer might ask you about the content of your supporting statement and the answers you might give.
Think about what you might need to read about before your interview – trust documents, recent important paramedic/NHS-related documents.
Think about questions you want to ask at interview.
How are you going to demonstrate your enthusiasm and commitment to the organisation?

There is quite a lot of preparation for an interview. If you are applying for jobs in more than one ambulance trust, you will be spending a lot of your time on preparation.

As the student response in Box 16.2 explains, there is usually not only a face-to-face interview, but also other tests. The information sent to you by your chosen NHS ambulance trusts prior to interview will provide more detailed information.

Box 16.2 What advice would you give to students prior to their paramedic interview?

📖 **Student paramedic response:** By the end of your programme – for me this was year 3 – you are getting fed up with filling out forms and writing personal statements, etc. so the application process can be a little tiring. Also, we had fitness tests to complete and advanced life support scenario assessments, as well as a panel interview.

Having made it so far, the thought of not getting a job offer at the end was a bit of a nightmare – I'd invested so much of my life into getting to that point and just wanted it all over. Fortunately, I passed all the tests and got the offer of a job. I felt like I'd won the lottery!

In the same way that the uni course interviewers are looking to see the type of person you are, not just the things you know, so the assessors on the interview day are looking for 'who you are', not simply that you've met the required standard for performing certain skills. Obviously you'll be nervous, but be yourself as far as you can. Yes, do your home-work, practise your skills and protocols till you can do them in your sleep, but show them the person you are. Examples of how you've developed as a person over your three years of paramedic education are just as relevant as examples of the clinical skills you've mastered.

🎓 **Academic response:** Your personal statement is a chance to let your personality and character shine through. Write from the heart and show how you have developed as a result of your education. At interview, just be yourself. You will be nervous, and the interview panel will allow for this. In my experience successful candidates have shown they have warm personalities. Ensure you prepare yourself with a good knowledge of the trust you are applying for too. There is nothing worse than being asked a question about the trust and having no clue as to the answer.

🚨 **Paramedic mentor/PEd response:** Be properly prepared! Everybody has their own thoughts on what you will be asked at inter-view. Think about what you need to know.

It isn't only about trust information, e.g. how many calls they attend. Interviewers want to know *you* and why *you* should have the position. What makes you better than other candidates? The panel will sit and listen to lots of candidates.

I would suggest doing a simple SWOT (strengths, weaknesses, opportunities, threats) analysis so you are more aware of yourself and think about how you will be a benefit to the organisation. Consider other aspects, the necessities, as I call them, that you need to know to do your job, e.g. confidentiality, equality and diversity. Be prepared for the practical aspects of an interview. Do you have a fitness test, are you prepared? Do you need additional clothing? Is there group work? How are you going to function in that group? Are there practical or theory-based exams? Make sure you know algorithms. Bring pens, paper and equipment with you, including your stethoscope. Examine your invitation letter and any other information sent through. Do not assume you know what they are looking for, make sure you *do* know what and who they are looking for.

The advice in Box 16.2 advises you to be yourself. This is hard to do at interview, but preparing and having a strategy on the interview day may help. Box 16.3 covers some main points. These may seem common sense, but at times of stress, simple things can be overlooked.

Box 16.3 Some interview tips about the face-to-face panel interview

- Arrive early.
- Dress professionally.
- Reread your supporting statement and highlight questions that you may be asked about it.
- Practise your responses to questions beforehand.
- Greet the interviewer formally (even if you know them).
- Do not sit down before the interviewer, unless given permission to do so.
- Shake hands on entering the room (if this seems appropriate) and smile.
- Try to let the interviewers see a bit of your personality, even if you are nervous.
- During interview, sit quietly, be attentive.
- No gum, phone calls or slouching.
- Ask appropriate questions about the organisation or specific job for which you are applying.

- Avoid a 'what can you do for me?' approach.
- Focus on your talents, interests and skills fit with the organisation.
- Answer questions as honestly and confidently as possible.
- Try to avoid answering a question by repeating it when you start giving your answer.
- Shake hands at close of the interview and thank the interviewers for their time.

This chapter has guided you through the process of applying for, and interviewing for, your first job as a paramedic. The comments provided by the contributors relate to their own experiences and thoughts. It is hoped that these provide an insight into the process, but fully investigate this for yourself, in relation to the ambulance trust that you want to work for. Good luck!

Once you have secured that paramedic position the support does not abruptly end, as Chapter 17 explains.

Suggested reading

Read all documents relating to the job you have applied for and the interview process. If anything is unclear, ask the trust or your university lecturers to see if they can help you.

Research any relevant trust or ambulance-related documents prior to interview.

Review your skills and make sure, if there are practical tests, that you know what to expect. Review relevant notes and texts about these skills or tests.

17 PRECEPTORSHIP

Prior to a period of preceptorship your employing NHS ambulance trust will usually provide an orientation period for new employees. Before discussing preceptorship, this chapter will examine the first few weeks of your employment.

Making the most of your orientation period

The orientation period may be called different things by NHS trusts, for example, induction or transition. For the purposes of this chapter the term 'orientation' will be used. Orientation involves raising awareness of the trust generally, reviewing policies, skills, procedures and mandatory training required by all employees. For paramedics who do not have their emergency driving course, this may also be included as part of their trust orientation. Box 17.1 explores feelings and advice relating to the orientation period that you may find useful.

> **Box 17.1 What advice would you give new registrants about their orientation to their NHS trust?**
>
> **Paramedic response:** Sitting in our trust orientation lectures, I couldn't help thinking about those old Battle of Britain war films where the new pilots who were about to face combat for the first time are being instructed on how to stay alive. The inevitability of being out on shift with 'paramedic' written on my shoulders loomed very large and I hoped I would last longer than the two-week life expectation of a Spitfire pilot. Whilst being scared of going out there for the first time, there is also a strengthening feeling of 'I just want to get on with it now. I'm not sure that another lecture will give me any more theoretical knowledge than I've already had drummed into me. I need to get out and do it for real.'

I guess you reach the point where you realise that the only way of gaining the confidence you lack is through experience on the job. It's scary and exciting at the same time.

🚨 **Paramedic mentor/PEd response:** You will usually undergo an orientation session/course on entering an ambulance trust. Don't be afraid to ask questions. You will find colleagues a good source of information; do not hesitate to ask them for help. Most people will only be too happy to give you a hand. Remember that although trusts do have differences, the work they do is fundamentally the same and you will have already had good experience of ambulance service culture on placement.

However long your period of orientation is, it may seem like an extension of your studies and you may feel like the paramedic in Box 17.1 who just wanted to get out there and do it for real. Or you may still be experiencing a wobble in your confidence. But once you have finished your orientation period you have a period of preceptorship to complete, where you will be supported, as the next section of this chapter explains.

𝒞 Refer to Chapter 15 for more guidance on improving your confidence in practice.

Preceptorship

This term may be new to you. It acknowledges that new registrants in any health-care profession will be safe and competent, but nonetheless novice clinicians, who will continue to develop their competence as part of their career development (Barrett and Nelson 2014). An official definition is provided by the Department of Health (2010).

Definition: Preceptorship

Preceptorship is 'a period of structured transition for the newly registered practitioner during which he or she will be supported by a preceptor, to develop their confidence as an autonomous professional, refine skills, values and behaviours, and continue on their journey of life-long learning' (Department of Health 2010: 11).

It is possible that even with the definition above, the preceptorship role is interpreted differently by organisations, preceptors or new registrants. It is therefore important to explore what preceptorship is not. See Table 17.1.

Table 17.1 What preceptorship is not

Preceptorship is not:
1. Intended to replace mandatory training programmes
2. Intended to be a substitute for performance management processes
3. Intended to replace regulatory body processes to deal with performance
4. An additional period in which another registrant takes responsibility and accountability for the newly registered practitioner's responsibilities and actions (i.e. not a further period of training)
5. Formal coaching (although coaching skills may be used by the preceptor to facilitate the learning of the newly registered practitioner)
6. Mentorship
7. Statutory or clinical supervision
8. Intended to replace induction to employment

Source: Department of Health (2010: 12).

It is important to note the differences between mentorship and preceptorship, as indicated by points 5 and 6 in Table 17.1. Preceptorship, as indicated by point 4 in Table 17.1, is not viewed as a way to meet any shortfall in pre-registration education, but as a transition phase for newly registered practitioners as they continue with their professional development. Barrett and Nelson (2014) explain that preceptorship provides an opportunity to build the practitioner's confidence in decision-making and further develop their competence for practice. In order for this preceptorship period to be successful, the preceptor is usually an established paramedic, with a minimum of 12 months of post-qualifying experience. In addition to experience, it is recommended that preceptors complete a programme with an HEI to develop their skills and knowledge of supporting newly qualified registrants (Gopee 2011).

What to expect from your preceptorship period

The process of preceptorship should be structured and form part of the orientation, induction and development of new staff, not necessarily just new registrants. Experienced paramedics who move from trust to trust may also be given a period of preceptorship, although this may vary in its duration or structure from that of a new registrant. The content of the preceptorship programme is usually planned in relation to the professional responsibilities of the paramedic and the needs of the employer, as per the guidance contained within the Department of Health (2010) preceptorship framework document. As with most things, it may not always be what you expected, as the responses in Box 17.2 explain.

Box 17.2 Was your period of preceptorship what you expected it to be?

Paramedic mentor/PEd response: I think preceptorship is heavily influenced by you as a professional. By this point you have successfully passed your studies, you have become a registered health-care professional and you have successfully landed yourself a job! So well done! This is your final chance to have direct support right beside you, so make the most of it. We were told all about preceptorship on our orientation to the trust and issued with a book to identify areas to cover during our preceptorship period. I personally found my preceptorship period invaluable. Using this opportunity to learn all you need to know about your new station, you can ask all those questions that you haven't yet asked. You are able to make those first decisions as a registered paramedic, which I found really quite scary, compared to student decisions, but know that there is still someone there to support you. You can iron out any concerns you have and know that other people have been exactly where you are, taking that first step. You are able to highlight areas you feel most confident in and areas you still wish to develop. I would say from the advice we were given about our preceptorship period from the university and from the ambulance services themselves, I had a very smooth transition from student to paramedic and utilised my time to the fullest, achieving all that I wished preceptorship to be.

📢 **Paramedic mentor/PEd response:** Many students think that gaining their paramedic qualification will add extra stress. For me the opposite was true – I found my job a lot less stressful as a paramedic than I ever did as a technician. For one, I had control over situations. Previously, I was forced to back down to the paramedic – even though I knew it was not good practice. I had also been given more skills to help my patients and did not have the stress of having to wait for paramedic back-up to treat my patients. The biggest challenge I found was not having the psychological safety net of another paramedic. The thing to remember here is that you may be lucky enough to be working with an experienced technician who, although not a paramedic, may have years of excellent experience for you to call on.

The Department of Health (2010) framework has been accepted as the foundation for preceptorship in the paramedic profession. The College of Paramedics (2014: 54) also recommends the following during the first six months following registration (see Table 17.2).

Table 17.2 Additional recommendations for the paramedic during the first six months following registration (College of Paramedics 2014: 54)

C6.6.12 Paramedics should not respond in isolation.

C6.6.13 During their first 150 hours post-registration, paramedics should have support from an experienced paramedic, with opportunities to access this support in their initial 12 months post-registration.

C6.6.14 Paramedics should not undertake supervision of a new member of emergency support staff or peer for at least 12 months following registration.

C6.6.15 A 24-hour advice line should be available to provide clinical support.

It is important that new registrants are aware of the College's recommendations and take advantage of the support available to them.

𝒞 Refer to Chapter 2 in relation to the value of support networks.

Reflection: points to consider

As a newly registered paramedic, what sort of support and help do you think a preceptor might be able to help you with?

This chapter has discussed the process of moving into employment. There are a variety of support networks available to you as a newly registered paramedic to be aware of and use to your advantage. Guidance and recommendations are available to NHS ambulance trusts relating to the employment of newly registered paramedics. This should ensure that all parties involved are aware of their responsibilities and ensure the smooth orientation and transition from student to registered paramedic.

Suggested reading

Barrett, K. and Nelson, L. (2014) Mentorship and preceptorship. In A.Y. Blaber and G. Harris (eds) *Clinical Leadership for Paramedics*. Maidenhead: Open University Press.

College of Paramedics (2014) *Paramedic Curriculum Guidance* (3rd edn). Bridgwater: College of Paramedics. Available at: https://www.collegeofparamedics.co.uk/downloads/Curriculum_Guidance_2014.pdf (accessed 18 February 2005).

Department of Health (2010) *Preceptorship Framework for Newly Registered Nurses, Midwives and Allied Health Professionals*. London: Department of Health.

Gopee, N. (2011) *Mentoring and Supervision in Healthcare* (2nd edn). London: Sage.

CONCLUSION

Your experience as a student paramedic will be as unique as you are as an individual. No two students have the same experiences. The theory taught to all students in your cohort has been the same, but how you each have interpreted it will have been different. Your clinical experiences may have dictated how you have focused your learning and developed your interests. To a large extent, students are in charge of their own destiny. It is now up to you!

INDEX

absence and sickness
  definitions and HCPC guidance, 86
accommodation and travel, costs of,
  31–2
'activist' learners, 57, 59
advocacy
  significance for patient care, 147–8
alcohol
  volatility and difficulty of obtaining
  consent of patients influenced by,
  88
ambulance emergency units
  significance as student placement
  venue, 128
ambulance services
  roles and importance in aiding and
  supporting student paramedics, 74
  types and significance for student
  placements, 126–9
  see also non-ambulance services
appearance and timekeeping, personal
  definition and HCPC guidance, 84–6
applications, job
  advice and requirements for
  successful, 207–12
assessors and assessment, student
  action when clash with mentor
  exists, 168–9
  process and players involved, 164–5
  significance of medical and surgical
  units for, 133
  types of assessment, 166–8
associate lecturers, 155–7
attitude, personal
  definition and HCPC guidance, 82–4
auditory learning, 60–1, 62–3

Barrett, K., 215
behaviour, professional

definition, parameters and guidance
  on, 79–93
blue-light driving course, 35–6
briefings, scenario
  significance as stage in simulation,
  113
  see also debriefs and debriefing
British Association for Immediate Care
  Schemes (BASICS), 128
burnout, 181–2

C1 driving category, 34–5
care, patient
  etiquette for homecare of patients,
  142–3
  extent of student paramedic
  responsibility for, 140–1
  fundamentals of, 145–8
  see also skills and attributes
  required e.g. advocacy;
  confidentiality, patient;
  commitment and dedication;
  communication; common sense;
  conscientiousness, academic;
  management and planning, self-;
  openness, personal; self-control
carers see families and carers
caring and empathy
  importance in defining successful
  students, 14
case studies
  choices surrounding level of
  academic programme, 25
  diversity of experiences in
  paramedic clinical practice,
  125–6
  example of independent study, 101
  joys and difficulties of advocating
  for patients, 147–8

linking theory to paramedic
practice, 120
paramedic feelings when solely
responsible for patients, 174, 175
patient confidentiality in differing
circumstances, 89–90
preparing for non-ambulance
service placements, 137–8
simulation as method of learning,
116–17
student experiences of debriefs,
160–1
student paramedic mentoring,
154–5
surprise element of crisis
experiences, 171
volatility and difficulty of obtaining
consent of alcohol influenced
patients, 88
vulnerability and ability to cope with
stress, 70–1
Casualties Union, 111
casualty, paramedic as
significance as element of
simulation,
113
centres, emergency control
significance as student placement
venue, 128
character, personal
definition and HCPC guidance, 81–2
cognitive behavioural therapy (CBT)
role in developing resilience, 184–5
colleagues
significance of student support
from, 161–3
College of Paramedics, 3, 26, 47, 50,
77–9, 126, 127, 132, 133, 154, 164,
203–4
commitment and dedication
importance as fundamental of
patient care, 145, 147
importance in defining successful
students, 14
common sense
importance in defining successful
students, 14

communication
importance as fundamental of
patient care, 145–6
significance for student paramedics,
16–17
compassion
importance as fundamental of
patient care, 145, 147
competence
importance as fundamental of
patient care, 145, 147
conduct, professional
definition, parameters and guidance
on, 79–93
confidence, loss of
experiences and causes of among
student paramedics, 197–9
confidentiality, patient
definition and HCPC guidance, 88–90
conscientiousness, academic
importance in defining successful
students, 14
consent, patient
definition and HCPC guidance, 86–8
content, curriculum
of paramedic programmes, 95–7
similarities in, 98–9
continuing professional development
definition, characteristics and
standards for, 202–3
conversations, paramedic-patient
tips for successful, 143–4
costs, accommodation and travel, 31–2
courage
importance as fundamental of
patient care, 145, 147
credits, academic
system of, 44–5
crises, situations of
case study of, 171
impact on student paramedics, 174–5
types faced by and student
responses, 170–4
culture, organisation
definition and implications for
student paramedics, 192–3
see also 'fitting in'

curriculum
content of paramedic programme,
95–7
similarities of, 98–9
see also guidance and support,
student; study
see also aids assisting e.g. materials,
guided study

day procedure units
significance as student placement
venue, 133
debriefs and debriefing
characteristics, importance and
benefits, 159–61
significance as stage in simulation,
113–14
see also reflection, personal
dedication and commitment
importance as fundamental of
patient care, 145, 147
importance in defining successful
students, 14
Denz-Penhey, H., 184
Department of Health, 149–50, 204,
216
departments, occupational health
role as venue for student support,
186
departments, paediatric
significance as student placement
venue, 133
departments, student support and
guidance
roles and importance in aiding
students through university,
74
development, clinical
student beliefs and responses
concerning, 9–10
see also environments; experiences,
clinical
see also factors hindering e.g.
finance, personal
see also qualities enabling
successful e.g. caring and
empathy; commitment and

dedication; common sense;
conscientiousness, academic;
management and planning, self-;
openness, personal; self-control;
skills, communication
driving
advantages, disadvantages of, and
courses aiding, 34–6
education
opportunities provided by
simulation, 115–18
use and importance of simulation,
108–14
educators, paramedic
value and importance for student
paramedic pathway, 152–5
see also specific e.g. mentors and
mentoring
emergency control centres
significance as student placement
venue, 128
empathy and caring
importance in defining successful
students, 14
employers and employment
advice and requirements for
applications, 207–12
considerations when applying for
first paramedic role, 205–7
considerations of whilst studying,
32–3
management and planning of
supernumerary, 52
possibility of supernumerary during
training, 47, 49
see also orientation, employment;
preceptorship
enactment, scenario
significance as stage in simulation,
113
environments
student beliefs and responses
concerning clinical, 8–9
see also specific e.g. homes, patient
ethics, professional
definition, parameters and guidance
on, 79–93

experiences, clinical
definition and interpretations of
'appropriate,' 13–16
importance of gaining, 18–19
see also development, clinical
see also features enhancing e.g.
caring and empathy;
communication; feedback;
transferable skills

families and carers
etiquette for care in homes of,
142–3
fundamentals of care for, 145–8
significance and importance of
student support from, 161–3
student paramedic responsibilities,
140–1
see also conversations, paramedic-
patient
feedback
significance as stage in simulation,
113–14
fees, university, 30–1
fidelity
significance in paramedic education,
110–11
finance, personal
importance for successful
paramedic studies, 8
see also particular e.g. costs,
accommodation and travel; fees,
university; transport, personal
'fitting in'
tips and advice from students about,
191–2
Fleming, N.D., 60–3
food
importance for mainlining
well-being, 67–8
formal assessments, 166
formative assessments, 166–8
Francis Inquiry and Report (2013), 17,
147, 148–9
friends
significance and importance of
student support from, 161–3

Galloway, J., 177–8, 179
Gopee, N., 177–8, 179
guidance and support, student
characteristics and variety of,
186–8
importance of available provision,
104–5
importance of families, friends and
colleagues, 161–3
roles and importance of universities
in aiding, 74
significance and importance of
accessing, 157–9
see also players involved e.g.
mentors and mentoring
see also types e.g. debriefs and
debriefing; networks and
networking
Guidance on Conduct and Ethics for
Students (HCPC), 77, 79–80, 81,
82–3

Hawkins, P., 178–9, 181
Health and Care Professions Council
(HCPC), 3, 23, 47, 48, 50, 76–8, 151,
202–3
homes, patient
etiquette for paramedic care in,
142–3
Honey, P., 56, 57–9

informal assessments, 166
informed consent, patient
definition and HCPC guidance, 86–8
injury and illness
importance of preventing, 64–73
significance of units for as
placement venues, 133
Institute of Health and Care
Development (IHCD), 36
interviews and selection
prior preparation for job, 209–12
process and alternatives for student
paramedics, 20–1

Jackson, D., 184
jobs see employers and employment

kinaesthetic learning, 60–1, 63
Kolb, D., 56–7

learners, student *see* students,
  paramedic
learning *see* education
lecturer practitioners
  definition and roles, 155–7
  roles and importance in aiding
  students through university, 74
life experiences
  importance in defining successful
  students, 14
link lecturers, 155–7
location, paramedic programme
  choices of, 26–7
  see also particular e.g. universities

management and planning
  of learning programmes, 50–3
  of study time, 53–6
management and planning, self-
  paramedic student regrets about,
  10–12
medical assessment units
  significance as student placement
  venue, 133
mentors and mentoring
  case study of, 154–5
  value and importance for student
  paramedic pathway, 152–5
  see also forms of e.g. debriefs and
  debriefing
  see also specific e.g. associate
  lecturers; lecturer practitioners;
  link lecturers
minor injury and illness units
  significance as student placement
  venue, 133
Murdoch, C., 184
materials, guided study
  definition, characteristics and
  use by student paramedics,
  102–4
  see also guidance and support,
  student
mini multiple interviews (MMIs), 20

money
  importance for successful
  paramedic studies, 8
  see also particular aspects e.g.
  costs, accommodation and travel;
  fees, university; transport,
  personal
Mumford, A., 56, 57–9

National Nursing Strategy for England,
  145
needs, learning support
  significance of available provision,
  104–5
Nelson, L., 215
networks and networking
  availability and significance of
  support, 27–9
  definition and HCPC guidance for
  social, 91–3
  role of support networks,
  186–7
Newman, R., 182
NHS Commissioning Board, 145
NHS England, 146–7
non-ambulance services
  characteristics, types and benefits
  of placements in, 132–5
  preparing for placement experience
  in, 135–9
non-emergency services
  significance as student placement
  venue, 128–9
non-maleficence
  significance in paramedic education,
  109

observation
  significance as element of
  simulation, 112–13
occupational health departments
  role as venue for student support,
  186
Open University, 23
openness, personal
  importance in defining successful
  students, 14

operating theatres
significance as student placement
venue, 133
organisations, culture of
definition and impact for student
paramedics, 192–3
see also 'fitting in'
orientation, employment
significance and advice regarding,
213–14
outcomes, learning, 53

paediatric departments
significance as student placement
venue, 133
Paramedic Curriculum Guidance
(College of Paramedics), 95,
132–3, 164, 217
Paramedic Evidence-based Education
Project, 26
paramedics
definition, context and career
pathway, 3–4
definition, parameters and guidance
on professional behaviour, 79–93
distinctive features of qualifications,
4
see also practice, paramedic;
registration, paramedic; students,
paramedic
participation
significance as element of
simulation, 112
patients
definition and HCPC guidance on
confidentiality of, 88–90
definition and HCPC guidance on
consent of, 86–8
etiquette for care in homes of,
142–3
fundamentals of care for, 145–8
student paramedic responsibilities,
140–1
see also conversations,
paramedic–patient
see also families and carers
patients, paramedics as

significance as element of
simulation, 113
Patients First and Foremost (Dept. of
Health), 149–50
periods, study
importance for successful
paramedic training, 6, 7
placements, student
characteristics, types and benefits
of non-ambulance service,
132–5
preparing for non-ambulance
service, 135–9
SETS relating to support on, 151–2
types of ambulance service, 126–9
see also factors impacting e.g. shift
work
see also players involved e.g.
mentors and mentoring
see also services e.g. guidance and
support, student
placements, supernumerary block
definition, characteristics and
possibility during training, 46,
49
management and planning of, 51
see also students, paramedic
planning and management
of learning programmes, 50–3
of study time, 53–6
planning and management, self-
paramedic student regrets about,
10–12
portfolios, student
development and use of, 201–2
post-traumatic stress disorder (PSTD),
180–2
practice, paramedic
diversity of experiences of, 125–6
ideas for study and during final year,
199–201
strategies for linking theory with,
118–21
see also locations e.g. placements,
student
see also factors impacting e.g. shift
work

preceptorship
  definition and characteristics,
    214–15
  expectations for process of, 216–18
*Preceptorship Framework for Newly
    Registered Nurses ...* (2010), 217
'pragmatist' learners, 60
preparation, academic
  importance of independent study,
    6, 7
  need for appropriate prior to
    paramedic studies, 5–6
professions and professionals, care
  current concerns with, 148–50
  see also specific e.g. paramedics
programmes, paramedic
  academic credit system involved,
    44–5
  clinical practice aspects, 45–50
  curriculum content, 95–7
  importance of exploration of
    university opportunities, 29–30
  levels of study, 24–6, 41–4
  location choices, 26–7
  management and planning of, 50–6
  significance of financial
    commitment, 30–4
  significance of learning styles, 56–63
  similarities of content, 98–9
  see also continuing professional
    development; guidance and
    support, student; preparation,
    academic; qualifications,
    paramedic; registration,
    paramedic; students, paramedic;
    study
  see also aids enhancing e.g.
    materials, guided study;
    portfolios, student
  see also forms e.g. guided study

qualifications, paramedic
  distinctive features of paramedic, 4
  extent of competition to obtain,
    19–21
  student beliefs and responses
    concerning, 9–10

  see also preparation, academic;
    programmes, paramedic
  see also factors impacting e.g.
    environments; finance, personal;
    transport, personal
questions and questioning
  significance as stage in simulation,
    113

'reflector' learners, 58, 59
reflection, personal
  significance for physical and mental
    well-being, 69–73
  see also debriefs and debriefing
registration, paramedic
  considerations and transition to
    acquiring, 197–218
  process and timing of application
    for, 201
  see also continuing professional
    development
  see also tools aiding e.g. portfolios,
    student
resilience
  characteristics of resilient
    individuals, 184
  definition and characteristics, 182–3
  student development of, 184–5
responses, student
  to crisis situations, 170–4
responsibility, patient care
  negotiation on extent of student
    paramedic, 140–1
Royal College of Surgeons, 111

scenarios
  significance as stage in simulation,
    113–14
selection and interviews
  prior preparation for job, 209–12
  process and alternatives for student
    paramedics, 20–1
self-control
  importance in defining successful
    students, 14
services, ambulance
  roles and importance in aiding and

supporting student paramedics, 74

types and significance for student placements, 126–9

shifts (work shifts)

characteristics, difficulties and pleasures of, 129–32

importance of coping and maintaining sleep, 64, 66–7

importance of health maintenance and illness prevention, 65, 67–73

shifts, supernumerary clinical

definition, characteristics and possibilities during training, 46–7, 48, 49

management and planning of, 51–2

see also students, paramedic

Shohet, R., 178–9, 181

sickness and absence

definitions and HCPC guidance, 86

simulation

definition, characteristics and experiences of, 107–8

elements, stages of and importance for learning, 112–14

opportunities presented for learning, 115–18

reasons for use in paramedic education, 108–12

types, 111

single response vehicles

significance as student placement venue, 128

sites, social networking

definition and HCPC guidance, 91–3

situations, crisis

case study of, 171

impact on student paramedics, 174–5

types faced by and student responses, 170–4

skills, communication

importance as fundamental of patient care, 145–6

significance for student paramedics, 16–17

skills, transferable

significance for student paramedics, 16–18

see also particular e.g. caring and empathy; communication

sleep

importance of maintaining, 64, 66–7

specialist operations units

significance as student placement venue, 128

Standards of Conduct, Performance and Ethics, 3, 4, 77, 86, 91, 92

Standards of Education and Training (SETs), 47, 95, 96, 98, 151–2

Standards of Proficiency (HCPC), 4, 77, 95, 97, 98

statements, job applications

advice for preparation of, 207–8

Stevenson, J., 17

stress

definition and symptoms, 179–80

sources of, 178

see also post-traumatic stress disorder; situations, crisis

structures, training programme

types and flexibility of, 46–7

see also particular e.g. employers and employment; placements, supernumerary block; shifts, supernumerary clinical

students, paramedic

current concerns with work of, 148–50

development and use of portfolios, 201–2

distinctive features of qualifications for, 4

feelings when solely responsible for patients, 174, 175

ideas for study and practice preparation in final year, 199–201

impact of crisis situations, 174–5

importance and interpretations of 'appropriate' experience, 13–19

interviews and selection, 20–1

popularity and extent of competition to become, 19–21

reality of roles of, 5–13

responses to crisis situations, 170–4
see also continuing professional
development; guidance and
support, student; placements,
student; preceptorship;
programmes, paramedic;
registration, paramedic
*see also elements of behavioural
roles e.g.* attitude, personal;
character, personal;
confidentiality, patient; consent,
patient; networks and networking;
reflection, personal; resilience;
sickness and absence;
timekeeping and appearance,
personal
see also elements of experience e.g.
assessors and assessment,
student; care, patient;
conversations, paramedic-patient;
lecturer practitioners; services,
ambulance
see also factors impacting e.g.
confidence, loss of; culture,
organisation; 'fitting in';
well-being, physical and
mental
see also outcomes e.g. employers
and employment; registration,
paramedic
studies, paramedic *see* programmes,
paramedic
study
definition, characteristics and use of
guided, 102–4
definition, characteristics and use of
independent, 99–102
ideas for paramedic practice and
during final year, 199–201
importance of independent for
successful training, 6, 7
see also continuing professional
development; guidance and
support, student; registration,
paramedic
see also tools e.g. portfolios,
student

styles, learning
types and significance of knowledge
of, 56–63
summative assessments, 166–8
support, student *see* guidance and
support, student
surgical assessment units
significance as student placement
venue, 133

'theorist' learners, 58, 59–60
theory, paramedic
strategies for linking practice with,
118–21
time
management and planning of
learning, 53–6
student regrets about self-
management of, 10–12
timekeeping and appearance,
personal
definition and HCPC guidance, 84–6
training, paramedic *see* programmes,
paramedic
transferable skills
significance for student paramedics,
16–18
see also particular e.g. caring and
empathy; communication
transport, personal
necessity for during study, 31–2
see also driving
travel and accommodation, costs of,
31–2
tutors, personal
roles and importance in aiding
students through university, 74

units, day procedure
significance as student placement
venue, 133
units, medical and surgical assessment
significance as student placement
venue, 133
units, minor injury and illness
significance as student placement
venue, 133

units, specialist operations
  significance as student placement
    venue, 128
universities
  importance of student visits to,
    29–30
  see also departments, student
    support and guidance;
    lecturer practitioners;
    students, paramedic;
    tutors, personal

vehicles, single response
  significance as student placement
    venue, 128
visual, auditory, reading, kinaesthetic
  (VARK) model of learning, 60–1,
    62–3
visual learning, 60-1, 62

well-being, physical and mental
  importance of maintaining, 64–73
work *see* employers and employment

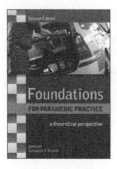

Foundations for Paramedic Practice
A theoretical perspective
2nd Edition

Amanda Blaber

ISBN: 978-0-335-24387-7 (Paperback)
eBook: 978-0-335-24390-7
2012

Foundations for Paramedic Practice is valuable to student paramedics studying within Higher Education. It differs from many existing texts in that it focuses solely upon the main theoretical subject's that student paramedics are required to study. The leading book is written by subject experts, many of whom are experienced paramedics working within Higher Education.

Key features include:

- New chapters on Specialist development roles
- Encourages the reader to reflect upon their practice experience
- Contains relevant case studies thorughout

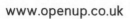
www.openup.co.uk

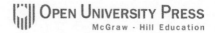
OPEN UNIVERSITY PRESS
McGraw · Hill Education